End the Food Confusion

End the Food Confusion

A Complete Guide to Good Nutrition

Sonia Jones ND

Zambezi Publishing Ltd

Published in 2008 by
Zambezi Publishing Ltd
P.O. Box 221 Plymouth, Devon PL2 2YJ (UK)
web: www.zampub.com email: info@zampub.com

British Library Cataloguing-in-Publication Data:
A catalogue record for this book is available from
the British Library

Typeset by Zambezi Publishing Ltd, Plymouth UK
Printed and bound in the UK by Lightning Source (UK) Ltd

(ISBN-10):   1-903065-72-0
(ISBN-13): 978-1-903065-72-3

135798642

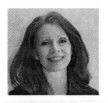

About the Author

Sonia is a qualified Naturopath, Reflexologist and Nutritional Therapist, who has been in professional practice for about fifteen years. She has studied and researched the effects of modern lifestyles and diets, and now specialises in chronic illness and holistic diet programs.

Having run very successful clinics in the UK and Malta, Sonia has now set up a clinic (www.thehavenspa.com) in a beautiful part of Panama, where she happily analyses health issues and develops not only appropriate solutions, but ways of preventing potential problems as well.

Dedication

I would like to express my gratitude to all the patients I have seen over the years who have encouraged me.

My thanks for love and support from my family Howard, Darren, Hanna, Malcolm and Else.

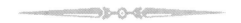

Contents

PART TWO
Good Eating

PART THREE
Weight Loss and Health

PART FOUR

In The Kitchen

PART 5

A to Z of Symptoms

PART SIX

Giving the Detox Process a Helping Hand

Foreword

Every paper and most magazines seem to include a page-filler on the subject of nutrition. The advice in one publication can conflict with the next, and one can't always be sure that the writers are actually qualified in nutrition. Is it any wonder that people are confused? Hence the title: "End the Food Confusion".

Sonia's book is subtitled "A complete guide to good nutrition", because it covers a wide range of subjects, and it doesn't simply harp on about one topic or climb onto the latest popular bandwagon.

"End the Food Confusion" is a fascinating read, full of information for those who want to eat well, and it is also very useful to those who advise others on dietary matters.

Sonia's principles of good nutrition can help us all to maintain a really good state of health and well being.

Sasha Fenton

Introduction

A Better State of Health

*"The lunches of fifty-seven years had caused his chest
to slip down into the mezzanine floor"*
P. G. Wodehouse: The Heart of a Goof

How many times have you heard the expression, 'You are what you eat'? We say it, we hear it, we read it, but how many of us stop to think what this actually means? When asked, most people will tell you they are healthy - viewing health as an absence of disease, because if we don't have a named disease then we must be healthy. Yet, on closer questioning, these very same people will tell you they have little or no energy, suffer frequent headaches, general aches and pains, mood swings and insomnia, to mention but a few forms of discomfort. The truth is that very few people experience a really good level of health. I seldom come across people who wake up in the morning with vigor and plenty of energy.

Look at someone who is healthy and note their energy levels, their clear eyes and their sparkle for life. Their skin glows and they are bubbling with enthusiasm. Bear in mind that I am not talking about the false energy that nicotine, caffeine, sugar or salt give us.

With a little know-how, you can also achieve a better state of health. Few of us have reached the point of no return, so it's never too late to consider changing.

Before you read on, I would like to ask you to write down everything you eat and drink during the course of a normal week. It will give you a very clear picture, maybe for the first time, of what's going on. In my experience, most people are not fully aware of precisely what they are eating and drinking until they see it all in writing. Once you have done this, put your notes away safely and return to them when you have finished reading this book.

Health

Unfortunately, most of us take our health for granted until something goes wrong. This is a shame, because prevention is always easier and better than cure. As the saying goes, 'You don't know what you've got until it's gone'. This is so true of our health.

Our needs for health are simple - fresh air, pure drinking water, sunshine and fresh, living food. I'm sure you would agree that these are the bare essentials of life. However, most people consider coffee, chocolate and bread essential to their well-being. I come across very few people who drink water on a regular basis, let alone eat much in the way of live, fresh, enzyme-rich foods.

I have heard people say that eating healthily is too expensive. Healthy foods don't have to be more expensive, but health care costs and medical tests can be very expensive. You can pay now or pay later. Of course, there are no guarantees. Eating healthy food doesn't guarantee you will never be sick, but it will cut down the odds and should reduce the severity of any illnesses. We can choose to eat nutrient-poor foods or nutrient-rich foods - both types of foods are easy to find. Nutrient-rich foods are real foods that have gone through little or no processing, unlike nutrient-poor foods. The foods I'm talking about have energy and a 'life force'. I am not talking about the energy that we call calories. I am referring to the foods that are full of enzymes.

Take two seeds, say sunflower seeds, boil just one of them, then plant both the seeds in the same fertile soil, water them and wait for them to germinate. Of course, only one of the sunflower seeds will burst into life due to the enzymes still being intact. The seed that was heated has had its enzymes destroyed, so it's unable to germinate and burst into life.

Quick fix

Most of us have been led to believe there is a quick-fix answer to most things. For instance, if we have a headache, then a painkiller will do the trick. Heartburn? What can be easier than an antacid? We turn the symptoms off and consider that the problem has vanished. Not so: the painkillers have not dealt with the cause of the pain, and as soon as the painkillers wear off, the pain will come back. In addition, we need to consider the consequences of taking such measures on a regular basis.

For instance, regular use of certain painkillers can adversely affect our liver function.

Toxins and Detoxification

To turn degeneration into regeneration, we must first detoxify. We need to identify where our toxins are coming from and then give the body the necessary tools for cleansing and repairing. Detoxifying is something we normally only contemplate once a year after Christmas as a New Year's resolution, having gorged ourselves on cake, chocolate, roast potatoes and more alcohol than usual. The truth is that our bodies need to detoxify on a daily basis. Waste products need to be dealt with regularly in order to prevent chronic conditions from developing.

Where do our Toxins Come From?

There are many toxins, which can attack our bodies from a number of sources:

1. Our bodies produce toxins as a natural by-product of metabolism.
2. Other toxins are consumed via our food and drink.
3. Social habits like smoking, alcohol and drugs introduce toxins into our bodies.
4. Our environment is full of hazardous toxins.
5. Toxins are occupational hazards, such as fumes, dust, moulds, sprays, cleaning chemicals, and so on.
6. Negative thoughts can produce unhelpful chemicals.

So, toxins are a way of life and none of us can escape them all. What we can do is give the body the best materials to deal with these toxins efficiently. For most of us, the opposite is true. We consume excessive amounts of fat, sugar, artificial sweeteners, chemicals and preservatives, refined foods, salt and stimulants. This is hardly a recipe for health and vitality. More like a slow suicide.

Some people have decided that one way around their poor food choices is to take vitamins and minerals in the form of a pill. We should note that vitamins and minerals are called supplements, as they supplement a healthy diet, so they should not be used instead of a healthy diet.

Manufactured vitamins and minerals are always second best; they are more difficult to absorb and utilize than the vitamins and minerals from food. Many compounds found in natural foods have not yet been researched and cannot be replicated and put into a capsule or tablet. Nature has provided nutrients in complex unique combinations.

Degeneration and Regeneration

This book will show you how to turn degeneration into regeneration. There are two major aspects to this program:

1. To remove the causes of ill health and degeneration.
2. To provide the body with all the right materials for health and vitality to enable the body to regenerate.

Symptoms

Most of us think of detoxifying as something that we do for a short period of time, maybe for three or four days but this is not so. The body should be given the opportunity to rid itself of its debris every day, as easily and simply as possible with the minimum of effort. Below is a list of some warning signs that we should not ignore. When these things occur, it's because our bodies are trying to tell us something:

- ~ Tiredness and fatigue
- ~ Putting on weight easily
- ~ Trouble losing weight
- ~ Cellulite
- ~ Bloating and wind
- ~ Dull and lifeless skin
- ~ Feeling run down
- ~ Acne, eczema, or psoriasis
- ~ Food intolerance
- ~ Constipation and/or diarrhea
- ~ Mood swings
- ~ Restlessness or irritability
- ~ Indigestion
- ~ Aches and pains
- ~ Headaches
- ~ Heavy periods
- ~ Sinus problems
- ~ Pre-menstrual syndrome
- ~ Palpitations

If you have some of these symptoms, you need to consider changing your lifestyle and you need to start giving your body the necessary tools for detoxifying. These are warning signals, as our body is trying to tell us that it's struggling. Don't ignore or leave these symptoms of degeneration, they will become more serious. A garden left to its own devices will soon become overrun with weeds. Most of us don't really appreciate that our health is something to nurture and cultivate regular ly.

You may have noticed the list above includes 'food intolerance' as a symptom. This is because food intolerance is a symptom of something else that might be going on. The causes of food intolerance will need to be investigated. I have come across many patients who have been given a huge list of foods to avoid, with little or no additional advice. Mostly, there has been no investigation into the cause of their food intolerance.

Many people are told that they are intolerant to wheat. These people often turn to gluten-free products that are found in every supermarket, and eat plenty of gluten-free biscuits (cookies), cakes and bread. These foods are still highly processed, often containing highly refined ingredients, like white cornstarch or white rice starch, refined processed fats and plenty of refined sugar. They are not a healthy alternative to good eating.

At the beginning of the twentieth century, about ten per cent of our food was processed and refined. By the middle of the century, it was about twenty-five per cent. Now, at the beginning of the twenty-first century, nearly ninety per cent of our food is refined and processed! This is worrying...

The word 'gluten-free' has become synonymous with health. This isn't always the case. What about people with celiac disease? They should also eat nutritious foods. In this book, you'll read about many highly nutritious and gluten-free whole grains and seeds. The recipe section will show you many wholesome nutrient-rich foods that are naturally gluten-free. They are not processed or expensive and they will contribute to your health.

It's no good eating gluten-free products that are highly refined, highly processed and that contain very few nutrients and almost no fiber. To add insult to injury, these are also expensive.

Our tendencies towards intolerance and allergies are the results of modern living. Refined and processed foods pass into the bloodstream in a way that wouldn't normally happen if our diets were full of natural whole foods. It has been discovered that refined sugars and flours directly inhibit the protective effect of white blood cells and cause enormous amounts of stress on both the pancreas and the adrenal glands.

Other causes of food intolerances could be a lack of certain minerals and/or a lack of certain enzymes that would normally break down toxins and food properly. There could be an imbalance of certain fats, causing a shortage of essential fatty acids that are needed for the production of certain prostaglandins. These are chemicals similar to hormones. Then there is what is referred to as a leaky gut. Anything that is wrong needs investigating, and the underlining problem needs to be rectified.

What is a 'Leaky Gut?'

It's estimated that the average person consumes about 15 pounds (about 7 kilos) of chemicals each year! That is a lot of chemicals.

Research has shown that some of these substances actually interfere with our digestive process and can change the permeability of our gastrointestinal tract (GI tract). Our small intestines need to be permeable enough to allow correctly digested particles to enter the blood stream, for transportation to the liver. The liver is like a processing plant and distribution warehouse. When the gut becomes too permeable, larger molecules pass into the bloodstream. These molecules, which are too large to be recognized as food, are then treated as foreign invaders, allergens that need destroying, and this causes a reaction in the body. So how does a 'leaky gut' come about in the first place, and how does it contribute to food intolerance in general? Here are a few suggestions:

~ Eating refined and processed foods and drinks
~ Drinking alcohol (more than just moderate amounts)
~ Medication; like antibiotics or the contraceptive pill
~ Nutritional deficiencies
~ The wrong acid/alkaline environment
~ Eating the same foods over and over again
~ Lack of certain enzymes

Overconsumption of the same foods will overwhelm and overtax our system. Out of hundreds of foods we can choose from, most people these days stick to about ten! Wheat is frequently at the top of the list. Think of all the foodstuffs that you eat several times a day, every day of your life, that contain wheat. Bread, biscuits, breakfast cereals, pizza, pasta, cakes, batter, pancakes and pies are made from wheat. There are plenty of other products that contain wheat, such as stock cubes, certain beers, whisky, sausages, most sauces and gravies, soy sauce, baking powder, Ovaltine and some ice creams. The list goes on and on.

The longer you continue to consume just a small variety of foods, the weaker your digestion and immune systems become. It's vitally important that you get as wide a variety of foods as you possibly can. Until recently, people varied their diets more, because foods were seasonal, so they couldn't eat the same thing every day, all year round.

This is the sort of diet that I tend to uncover during an individual case study, and it's frequently eaten throughout the year.

Breakfast
~ White bread toast with margarine and marmalade
~ Bran flakes with milk and sugar
~ Two cups of coffee each with sugar and milk
~ Orange juice (not freshly squeezed)

Mid-morning Break
~ Coffee or tea with sugar and milk
~ Two biscuits, and sometimes potato crisps or chocolate

Lunch at Work
~ Sandwich or roll (generally made from white flour), with cheese, ham, salami or tuna, maybe with a little lettuce tomatoes and cucumber.
~ Coffee with sugar and milk

Mid-afternoon Break
~ Chocolate or biscuits
~ Tea or coffee, sugar and milk

Evening Meal
~ Pasta with tomato sauce from a jar, or
~ Frozen pizza, or
~ Chicken with potatoes and peas, or
~ Fish in breadcrumbs with oven chips, frozen peas and fresh carrots that have been boiled, and the water thrown away
~ Coffee with sugar and milk

~ Chocolate or crisps, or maybe cake or something sweet, like
    chocolate mousse or processed fruit yogurt

Sunday Lunch
~ Roast meat with vegetables (boiled, water thrown away)
~ Roast potatoes, sometimes with bought Yorkshire pudding
Plus
~ Three pieces of fruit a week
~ Several cokes or soft drinks a week
~ A little water
~ Some alcohol

Our most precious possession should be our health. You wouldn't think so, looking at the average diet above. If you owned a very expensive racehorse, you would make sure everything it ate contributed to and enhanced its health, so it would look its best and, of course, perform at its best. We would give the horse the high performance fuel (good nutrition) to win races. We, however, expect our bodies to run the course of daily life on poor quality, nutrient-deficient, highly processed food, so it's no surprise that we are tired long before we reach the finishing post.

This book will help you to avoid the pitfalls of the modern diet.

In *Part One*, I shall examine the mechanisms employed by our bodies to process the foods we eat.

Part Two describes the foods themselves and how to get the maximum goodness from them.

In *Part Three*, I shall look at weight loss - how to achieve it permanently, and the obstacles you could meet on the way.

Part Four, In the Kitchen, provides recipes and advice on the properties of the herbs and spices that are used to flavor your food. This should give you a basis for adapting your general diet to include all you need for a healthy body.

You will find in *Part Five* a useful A - Z of symptoms, problems and situations and the appropriate dietary ways of addressing them.

The detox process is examined in *Part Six*, with advice on making it really work for you.

Finally, the *Glossary* explains the commonly used words and phrases used in this book. I hope that, by the time you have read my book, you will find that it's possible, and easy, to arm yourself with the naturopathic know-how to stay younger, healthier and slimmer.

Part One

Digestion

Chapter 1

Enzymes

"The discovery of a new dish does far more for the happiness of mankind than the discovery of a new star"
Anthelme Brillat-Saverin: Physiologie du Gout

Enzymes are needed for every chemical action and reaction in the body and metabolic enzymes run our system, encompassing our organs, tissues and cells. Without enzymes, there is no life and no movement. Enzymes are vital to our health.

What is an Enzyme?

Each enzyme performs a specific job within the body. Some are involved in digestion, while others aid detoxification or are needed for building new bones or skin. Just about every process needs enzymes. Any machine is lifeless until the batteries have been installed or the electricity has been switched on. It's the enzymes in our body that make things happen; otherwise, we too would be lifeless. An enzyme activates a reaction. Life cannot exist without enzymes. There are a huge variety of different enzymes and each one is busy doing its specific job. For instance, forming urea, aiding the immune system, helping in fertilization or transporting oxygen around the body. I could go on and on … Enzymes act upon substances by changing their original identity. Each enzyme has a specific job to do, otherwise there would be chaos.

It's important to understand that enzymes are extremely important to our health. Any deficiencies can cause us to age quickly and possibly suffer chronic diseases earlier or more severely. Enzymes break down toxic substances so that the body can eliminate them from our systems before they cause too much destruction and degeneration.

Where Do Enzymes Come From?

Our body can manufacture enzymes or they can come from our food. Although the latter statement is correct, most of us choose to eat food that is dead: that is to say, void of enzymes. What do I mean by dead food? These are foods that don't contain enzymes and contain little in the way of nutrients that would enable the body to make its own. The problem with enzymes is their sensitivity to heat. Cooking destroys them. So canning, frying, roasting, pasteurizing and so on, completely destroy the enzymes in our food.

Most foods people choose to eat are highly processed, such as white bread, biscuits, pizzas, cakes, pies, most breakfast cereals, etc. These foods have had their enzymes destroyed and their nutrients and fiber removed during the manufacturing process. Each time we eat such 'empty calories' our bodies have to find the enzymes and nutrients to digest these foods, causing a deficit somewhere inside ourselves. These foods leave us deficient in many ways. As time goes on the situation gets worse.

There are three categories of enzymes:
    Metabolic enzymes
    Digestive enzymes
    Food enzymes

All food must be broken down into simpler molecules by enzymes. The more enzymes we get from our food the less our system has to manufacture, borrow or steal from other activities within our bodies. The enzymes provided by the food we eat aid in their own digestion, leaving our own reserves to get on with other metabolic jobs that are vital to our health.

It has been found that young people have greater reserves of enzymes in their tissues compared to older people. In general, when a young person eats cooked foods there is a greater activity of enzymes than in an older adult. Have you ever wondered why we end up with digestive problems as we age? As our enzymes become depleted over the years, and as we continue to eat 'dead food', our digestive system struggles. The gradual depletion of enzymes means that most of our food isn't being digested properly. This situation, along with eating nutrient-poor foods, can lead to all sorts of chronic problems. Dead food isn't just void of enzymes, but also lacking in vitamins, minerals and fiber.

Studies have shown low levels of enzymes in diabetics. The pancreas is the organ that produces insulin and digestive enzymes. People suffering with liver problems have also been found to have low levels of digestive enzyme activity.

It's common today to find people living on stimulants. Every time the metabolism is falsely stimulated with things like caffeine, high-protein diets, sugar and so on, enzymes and nutrients are spent and our reserves are slowly used up. A false energy is experienced but eventually we become fatigued, until we take more of these stimulants, and so a dependency develops. We end up needing more and more of them to feel normal and this leads to premature ageing.

The high-protein diets so popular today are very stimulating and they can cause damage when the diet consists of more protein than the body needs. The by-product of protein is urea, which is a diuretic. This causes the kidneys to excrete extra fluids along with extra minerals in a situation where most people are already dehydrated and mineral deficient.

Vitamins and minerals depend on enzymes, while enzymes depend on vitamins and minerals. Nature has provided foods that are rich in both enzymes and vitamins and minerals. The speed of the metabolism is determined by the activity of the enzymes. During times of exercise and acute disease (especially fevers and infections), enzymes and nutrients are used up much faster than usual. Anything that increases heat in the body will speed up enzyme activity. As you would expect, enzyme activity also goes up during digestion.

There is a direct relationship between our enzyme reserve and the health of our immune system. The better our enzyme reserve, the more easily our immune system can cope with everyday battles - of which there are many.

White blood cells are responsible for seeking out and destroying foreign invaders that manage to infiltrate our blood and lymph. Studies have shown that these white blood cells have proteolytic, amylolytic and lipolytic enzymes similar to those produced by the pancreas for digestion. These enzymes break down proteins, fat and carbohydrates that have managed to get into the blood stream, thus dealing with them before they cause too much havoc or destruction in our system.

The system will not work properly where there is a leaky gut, as this allows larger food molecules to pass through the wall of the intestines and into the blood stream. These larger molecules of fat, protein and carbohydrates are seen as foreign invaders, causing our immune system to use up large amounts of its enzyme reserves. Why are these larger molecules seen as foreign invaders? Basically, they are not small enough for the body to make use of them, so the body tries to rid itself of them by attacking them.

Nothing can take place in the body without energy, and energy cannot be produced without enzymes. Enzymes cannot be produced without enough vitamins and minerals, often sadly lacking in our normal diets. Life itself requires a constant supply of enzymes. Is it any wonder that we begin to generally feel tired, given our typical diet? Our cells can only reap the benefits of the proteins, carbohydrates, and fats we ingest each day with the help of enzymes.

After a cooked meal, our white blood cell count goes up considerably as the body produces much-needed enzymes. However, when we eat raw foods, there is no such substantial increase in our white blood count. Raw foods bring with them plenty of their own enzymes, so our immune system does not need to produce extra enzymes to support digestion. A good working digestive system is vital to our health.

To increase your energy levels and dramatically improve your general health you need enzymes and co-enzymes (vitamins and minerals). The food that provides enzymes also provides co-enzymes. Dead foods are not only void of enzymes but they also lack the co-enzymes that we need for health and vitality.

Our first priority is to get the good quality materials that our factories need, and this is nutritious food. Secondly, the factory needs machinery that is in good working order and this is also true of our digestive systems. The best diet is of little value if the digestive system cannot break down food into components that the body can use. Thirdly, enzymes are what make the digestive system work, so we provide either enzymes or the necessary nutrients so that the body can make its own, just as a real factory needs fuel to make the machinery work.

Basically, we eat three types of food: proteins, carbohydrates and fats. For the digestion of these foods there are three basic groups of digestive enzymes: protease, or proteolytic enzymes that break down proteins, amylase, or amylolytic enzymes that break down starches (carbohydrates), and Lipase, or lipolytic enzymes that act on breaking down fats.

1. Proteolytic enzymes are broken down by amino acids, of which there are about twenty-two. Nine of these are called 'essential'. The body cannot make them, so they need to be provided by the diet.
2. Amylolytic enzymes break down carbohydrates.
3. Lipolytic enzymes break down fats that are called lipids.

Enzyme Inhibitors

There are many things in our environment that can affect enzyme activity.

Pesticides, including insecticides, herbicides and fungicides inhibit enzymes. They were first developed for use as nerve gas in WWII and they are now used to control pests. Fruit and vegetables are sprayed many times during their growing season. It's advisable to wash your fruit and vegetables thoroughly before you consume them, buy organic produce, or as a last resort peel your fruit and vegetables.

Salt and sugar. As you would imagine, salt and sugar inhibit activity. Both have been used for hundreds of years to preserve food and stop it spoiling.

Heavy metals like lead and mercury can inhibit enzymes. Lead can be found in canned foods, as some countries still use lead solder on the tins. Lead from petrol used to be a big problem. Old paint in old houses will have lead in it and if it's green, it may contain arsenic! Some metallic water pipes are soldered with lead solder, which can leach out into our drinking water. Mercury occurs naturally in most foods. These levels are not normally a problem, except where seafood is concerned, depending on which seas they are fished from. It can also be found in gray amalgam tooth fillings. This may surprise you, but mercury can be found in many prescription drugs! It was used as a treatment for syphilis, and when the patient went mad, it was hard to tell whether it was the disease or the treatment that caused the problem! Remember the Mad Hatter in Alice in Wonderland? Hatters used mercury in the production of hats. The constant touching and smoothing enabled the mercury to enter the hatters' systems through their skin and it eventually sent the poor men off their heads. The same thing happened to dentists who chose to wear sandals in the summer, as their toes came into contact with the beads of mercury that dropped down or lay around on the floor.

Food additives. There are thousands of them. They are used by the food industry to make food more palatable and to give foodstuffs a longer shelf life by using substances that improve texture, enhance flavor or improve the color. It's a big business. It's estimated that the average person eats several pounds of these chemicals each year. Who knows what long-term health hazards they bring? Individual food additives and chemicals have been researched, but the chemical cocktails that are consumed on a regular basis over a longer period are another matter altogether.

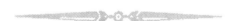

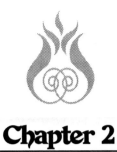

Chapter 2

The Digestive Process

"We lived for days on nothing but food and water"
W. C. Fields: attributed

Taste

The tongue has taste buds for sweet, salty, sour and bitter sensations. Each type of taste bud is located in a different part of the tongue, and taste is greatly enhanced by the aromas of the food reaching the receptors in the nose. This is why we have trouble tasting our food properly when we have a cold, because we can't smell our food.

A deficiency of zinc can affect our ability to taste food properly. There are also drugs and diseases that can affect our sense of taste and smell, as does smoking and ageing. If we don't taste our food properly, there is a danger of overcompensating with more salt than is good for us. If we are accustomed to eating processed foods, natural foods can taste quite bland at first, because our taste buds are attuned to the high levels of salt in processed foods.

Mouth

Chewing properly is of vital importance. Here, enzymes in our saliva mix with our food and begin to work on it. This is particularly so in the case of carbohydrates. Chewing increases the surface area of our food, making it easier for our enzymes to do their job. Chewing also tells the pancreas and gall bladder to get ready to go to work. So, if you chew your food well, it gives your whole digestive system a better chance. Besides, it would be very difficult to swallow if we didn't chew and produce saliva to act as a lubricant. Many people confess to gulping down their food and hardly stopping to chew. It's a difficult habit to get out of and will need a conscious effort to overcome.

No matter how old or young you are it's important to look after your teeth. If your teeth are uncomfortable, painful, broken or missing, it's more difficult to chew food properly. Even if you feel you have no dental problems, regular check-ups are advisable, as prevention is always better than cure. However, for most people, the problem isn't their teeth, it's a lack of time and eating on the run.

These are some of the things you need to consider when you eat.
   Don't eat:
   ~ while standing
   ~ while reading
   ~ if you are angry
   ~ while watching television
   ~ while on the phone
   ~ while working.

Concentrate on what you are eating, chew well and savor it. In truth, few people pay attention to how much they have eaten or to what they have eaten, as they are too busy doing something else. The small amount of extra time needed is well worth the investment, it will make a big difference to your digestion and ultimately to your health. It only takes a little extra time to eat properly.

While I am on the subject of chewing and eating, I suggest that you don't drink a lot of water with your meals. I am always telling people to drink more water, but not with meals. The water can dilute your digestive enzymes - and this is not a good thing, especially if you already have digestive problems. Drink some water half an hour before a meal, as this will encourage digestion. After you have eaten, wait an hour before you drink some more water.

The chewed food then enters the stomach where the lining of the stomach secretes hormones, enzymes and hydrochloric acid. The lining of the stomach secretes between one to two liters a day! Have you ever wondered why the stomach doesn't digest itself? This is due to the fact that it has a very thick layer of protective mucus.

What Will You Find In Your Stomach Juices?

Pepsin, which breaks down proteins. The stomach lining produces several types of pepsinogens, which are dormant until they are mixed with hydrochloric acid, at which point these form pepsin. If you don't have enough hydrochloric acid, the pepsinogens cannot be activated into pepsin, making protein digestion more difficult.

Hydrochloric acid is produced by the parietal cells in the stomach lining. Besides helping to break down proteins, it helps us to absorb minerals, especially calcium and iron. It also does a very important job of killing bacteria, fungus, etc. Our hydrochloric acid levels drop as we get older. It would appear that people with blood group A have lower levels of this acid than people with blood group O.

Rennin helps the milk to curdle and it adapts the protein Casein to make it easier for us to digest. It also helps to release calcium from milk. This also decreases with age.

Gastric lipase splits down fats.

Amylase. The stomach takes over from the saliva in continuing to break down carbohydrates.

Intrinsic factor. Without this, we cannot absorb Vitamin B12, and this causes pernicious anemia. Pernicious anemia isn't the same as the anemia caused by an inability to store iron.

The Digestive Process

Food will stay in the stomach for anything from one to five hours. The time varies depending on how much fat and protein is in the stomach. Fresh fruit eaten on its own doesn't take much time at all. Our *stomach* churns our food into a pureed-soup like consistency called chyme. Once chyme leaves the stomach, it enters the *small intestine*, which is twenty-two feet long!

When the chyme enters the *duodenum* (the first part of the small intestines), which is ten inches long (0.3m), hormones rush to the *pancreas* and the *gall bladder*. The pancreas produces about 2.5 liters of pancreatic juice a day.

The first thing that must happen is the production of a substance rich in sodium carbonate that will neutralize the stomach acid. This is because the lining of the duodenum cannot cope with such high acidic levels, as these would have a very corrosive effect. This is how duodenal ulcers can develop.

A hormone is released which signals the pancreas to release its digestive enzymes - amylase, lipase and three proteases. As we already know, these digestive enzymes further break down carbohydrates, fats and proteins.

The gall bladder will have released *bile salts*, breaking down fat into smaller parts and allowing the lipase enzymes to do their job more efficiently. Bile is a greenish-yellow colored fluid that contains cholesterol, fatty acids, lecithin, bilirubin and bile salts, and is produced by the liver. The bile salts are important to digestion. They emulsify fats by lowering the surface tension, allowing large particles to be broken down into tiny ones. Bile salts also help with the absorption of fatty acids from the intestinal tract.

Bile gets its color from the pigment called bilirubin, which come from spent and worn-out red blood cells that are removed from the blood stream for disposal. A good working *liver* and gall bladder are very important to the digestion and absorption of fat. I hear you say, I don't want to absorb fat. Oh, yes, you do; some fats are essential to health and weight maintenance. (More on this subject later).

The *jejunum* (the second part of the small intestine) is three feet long (1.3m), and this is where most of the absorption takes place. Enzymes play a vital role in the process of absorption from the small intestine into the blood stream.

In the *ileum* (the third part of the small intestine), which is five feet long (1.6m), bile salts and B12 are absorbed.

The *large intestine* or *colon*; by the time the food has reached here, most of what was worth using will have already been absorbed. The large intestine is about five feet long. Though the entire digestive tract contains bacteria, this is where the majority of bacteria can be found. They produce enzymes that continue to work on the rest of the digestive process. At this point, water is reabsorbed, and the longer the waste remains in the large intestine, the more water is removed. Therefore, the longer the waste remains in the large intestine, the harder the stools become and the more toxins are re-absorbed.

Gastrointestinal Tract

The mouth, esophagus, stomach, small intestines and large intestine down to the anus are collectively known as the gastrointestinal tract - GI tract for short. The liver, pancreas and gall bladder work with the GI tract, but are not actually part of it. The pancreas and the gall bladder have ducts that connect to the GI tract, allowing both the glands' digestive enzymes and other products to enter directly into the duodenum. Along the GI tract are regulating valves that keep each stage of digestion separate.

If the valve between the top of the stomach and the bottom of the esophagus doesn't remain properly closed, we could experience heartburn. The stomach content is very acidic, and when it comes into contact with the sensitive lining of the esophagus, it will cause pain. On the odd occasion, it can be so bad that sufferers can think they are having a heart attack. If the valve at the bottom of the stomach isn't working properly it might leak out its acidic contents and cause erosion in the duodenum causing pain and duodenal ulcers.

Food is propelled along the GI tract by contracting waves of muscle action known as peristalsis. The stomach has three layers of muscles that are circular, diagonal and longitudinal. They contract the stomach in different directions to mix the food, a little like a cement mixer.

Below is a very brief insight into the many nutrients needed by the digestive system to function properly:

Stomach:	Vitamin A, vitamin B complex, and zinc
Large intestine:	Vitamin E
Liver:	Vitamin C and B complex
Gallbladder:	Lecithin

These nutrients are often missing in processed and refined foods, but can be found in natural whole foods.

What Can Go Wrong?

There are many conditions that can interfere with digestion, such as trauma, stress, illness, chemicals, certain foods and depression.

We are all born with genetic weaknesses of one description or another. For some it can be a weak circulation, and for others it may be a weak digestive system. This does not mean that we can do nothing to help ourselves because whatever weaknesses we are born with, we can make improve or inflame the situation, depending on the lifestyle we choose.

This becomes even more of a problem as we age, as the quality and quantity of our digestive juices naturally decline with age. We can speed up the ageing process or we can slow it down: the choice is entirely ours.

We can provide the body with the things it needs or we can leave it struggling. Ageing is inevitable but chronic suffering is not. The good news is that much of the cure is within our control.

To improve our digestion we need enzymes and co-enzymes (such as vitamins and minerals). Poor nutrition puts a dreadful strain on the digestive system and immune system.

Heartburn and indigestion are very common problems these days, as the huge sales of antacids will confirm. They are one of the biggest selling over-the-counter medications.

There are certain foods and drinks that can increase the likelihood of acid reflux from the stomach up to the esophagus. Large meals, too much fat, alcohol, coffee (even decaffeinated), tea, fizzy drink, orange and chocolate will all lower the pressure of the sphincter muscle. The same is true of certain medications. There are a vast number of people using antacids of one description or another on a regular basis to help counteract acidity.

What do antacids do? Some antacids reduce stomach acidity so that it burns less. Others reduce stomach acid secretion so there is less lying around in the stomach to cause problems. The problem is that we need normal amounts of strong stomach acid to digest food properly. Lowering secretion or reducing stomach acidity on a regular basis could impair digestion in the long run, setting up all sorts of problems for the future. I am not referring to the odd occasion, such as Christmas or some other holiday when you eat far too much, but to regular use.

Henry D Janowitz MD, formerly Head of the Division of Gastroenterology, now Clinical Professor of Medicine Emeritus at the Mount Sinai School of Medicine, suggests that taking regular substantial amounts of aluminum-containing antacids can negatively influence the calcium in our bones.

So, What Are The Alternatives?

Experiment.
Maybe only one or two of these foods upset you, so avoid all of them for a few days and then gradually reintroduce them one at a time and wait at least twenty-four hours before introducing another food from the above list.

Being overweight increases physical pressure on the stomach, and this can force acid up into the esophagus. That is why heartburn is so common among pregnant women. If you are overweight, it's worth considering losing weight for this, as well as many other health reasons.

Smoking not only relaxes the valve at the top of the stomach, but it also increases stomach acid secretions.

More Digestion-Related Ailments

Diverticulitis

This is a relatively common condition found in the small or large intestine. Small pouches appear in the lining of the large intestine. These pouches become filled with waste products, becoming infected and causing pain. Symptoms are diarrhea and constipation, tenderness, bloating and feeling the need to go to the toilet the whole time.

To prevent this condition it's important to eat foods that are naturally high in fiber; these foods will also provide the necessary nutrients to maintain a healthy intestinal lining.

However, if you have diverticulitis, then a diet high in 'soluble fiber' is recommended, such as cooked oats, lentils, fresh fruit and vegetables in general. It's very important not to eat 'wheat bran' in its concentrated form - it's an insoluble fiber and far too harsh, and will cause irritation to an already inflamed intestinal lining. Steam vegetables lightly; this will soften them enough to prevent irritation.

Grind nuts and seeds. Linseeds/flaxseeds have mucilaginous properties so they will help to soothe the lining of the intestines. 'Mucilaginous' means they will go slimy when moistened, which is the perfect constituency for an irritated intestine. Flax/linseeds also contain anti-inflammatory compounds, helping to calm down inflammation. Also, the high fiber content of these seeds will speed up the transition of waste matter, which is so vital to the treatment of this condition. Take plenty of foods rich in vitamin C, such as fresh fruit (but not oranges, as they encourage inflammation).

Hiatus Hernia

Hiatus Hernia is a condition where the stomach lining bulges out into the chest area, causing pressure where food can back up the esophagus.

Causes vary: being middle-aged and overweight, being pregnant, lifting heavy objects or having a persistent cough. Chronic constipation can cause the need to strain while passing hard stools.

Symptoms can vary a lot from person to person; some experience no symptoms and the condition is only discovered after an x-ray for something else. A very common symptom is feeling a little uncomfortable under the breastplate after eating. Then there are the more severe symptoms of pain and burning, causing esophageal ulcers in the long run. For some, symptoms only appear at night or get worse once they lie down in bed.

Read the sections in this book on heartburn, constipation and/or losing weight.

If you are one of those whose symptoms are worse at night, try:
a)   more pillows
b)   raising the head end of the bed with some books
c)   eating smaller meals at night, and
d)   having nothing to eat or drink for three hours before bedtime.

Hemorrhoids

Most people call this condition piles. They are swollen and often painful veins around the anus. In reality, hemorrhoids are varicose veins that can be internal or external. There can be bleeding, which is bright, red and not part of the waste matter - in other words, the blood isn't mixed in with your stools, it's separate. The blood is on the toilet paper or in the water of the toilet bowl. There can be itching, pain, or discomfort.

What are the causes? Women often suffer this condition after giving birth, due to all the straining. Chronic constipation, being overweight, inherent weakness, lack of exercise and a job where heavy lifting is required can encourage hemorrhoids. After the age of 50, the condition is quite common in developed countries, due to our poor diets that lack fiber.

A complete change to a diet of whole foods is very important, as is making sure you are getting enough hydrating drinks. Include buckwheat on a regular basis; this grain/seed is a rich source of rutin, which helps to strengthen veins. Check out the recipe section, where you will find ideas on cooking with buckwheat. You can also buy soba noodles made from 100 per cent buckwheat, but always read the label as some brands add other ingredients.

Make juices that are high in vitamin C; just about any vegetable and fruit mixture can be used. Vitamin C strengthens connective tissue.

Linseeds are a must for this condition, as their mucilaginous effect can lubricate the intestines, making it much easier to pass a motion without straining. Place two tablespoons in a bowl and cover them with about four times the amount in water. Leave to soak overnight, and in the morning, they should be soft and slippery. If not, add more water next time. Add to your porridge (after it has been cooked) or to natural yogurt.

IBS (Irritable Bowel Syndrome)

IBS is a very common condition that can affect any age from childhood to adulthood. However, it's more common between the ages of 20 to 50 and affects men and women equally. IBS is a fairly vague term to describe a number of symptoms that vary from person to person. The main symptoms are periods of constipation alternating with periods of normal bowel movement or diarrhea. Some people experience pain, which is relieved by passing a motion. There is bloating and flatulence. In some cases, there can be nausea, indigestion and heartburn.

From a naturopathic point of view, there are several causes; the situation can be greatly improved and in some cases, completely cured, with a totally natural approach.

First, it's very important to have some tests done to exclude the possibility of a more serious problem, such as Crohn's disease, colitis, gall bladder disease or polyps. Generally, though, diet and stress seem to be the main problems for IBS sufferers.

The key is a diet rich in magnesium-containing foods like fish, nuts, beans, seeds and green vegetables. Cook with herbs that feed the nervous system, like rosemary, thyme, basil and nutmeg, and drink mint tea. Oats are a very good nerve tonic. Ground flax/linseeds would be very good. Eat natural yogurt on a regular basis to encourage the correct bowel flora. Avoid all forms of white flour products. Are you drinking enough hydrating drinks?

Also, try some form of relaxation. I can hear what you are thinking. When people hear me say relaxation they think it means doing nothing, but this is definitely not the case - doing nothing can be stressful. I mean take a walk with a friend, or find a hobby you enjoy, do anything that will take your mind off your daily hassles. I have found so many people with this condition are very anxious and always stressed. You need some rest and relaxation.

Peptic and Duodenal Ulcers

Ulcers can appear in the stomach (peptic ulcers) or in the first part of the small intestine (duodenum). The pain from duodenal ulcers could be described as a little like heartburn. The valve at the top of the stomach allows acid to seep up into the esophagus, causing pain in the chest area. There is also a valve at the bottom of the stomach that can allow acids to seep out into the delicate duodenum. This acid causes erosion of the intestinal lining and hence ulcers. Under normal circumstances, when the valve of the stomach opens and allows the contents to continue their journey, the pancreas produces buffering agents to neutralize the acidity and prevent damage and pain in the lining. If your diet and lifestyle regularly cause an overproduction of stomach acids your pancreas will not produce enough buffering agents, eventually causing erosion and hence pain in the duodenum.

There are several causes - bacterial infection, prolonged stress, smoking, large consumption of tea and/or coffee, orange juice, alcohol and any fizzy drinks, especially coca-cola type drinks. If you are blood group O, you are more likely to suffer from ulcers than the other blood groups. 'O blood types' naturally produce more stomach acids than 'A blood types'.

The helicobacter infection will need treating with a course of antibiotics. Remember, when you have finished the course of antibiotics, to take some pro-biotics to help recolonize the intestines with some friendly bacteria (the good guys).

It's important while trying to heal your ulcers, to give up all the drinks mentioned above as they encourage the overproduction of acid. Drink one large glass of freshly-made cabbage juice twice a day. Cabbage is high in Vitamin U, which gets its name from the fact that it helps to heal ulcers. If you have a thyroid problem don't drink cabbage juice, as it could further affect its function.

For a flaxseed/linseed infusion, put 2 or 3 teaspoons of seeds into a mug, pour boiling water over them and leave for about 10 to 15 minutes. Drink this in the morning and in the evening. This infusion will be mucilaginous and certainly help to soothe the lining of the digestive tract. You could also put the seeds into a mug, fill it with cool water and leave it overnight.

You will need to take a good look at your lifestyle - find some time for a regular massage, acupuncture, reflexology, yoga or tai chi. Giving up caffeine will greatly reduce your anxiety and the stress on your adrenal glands. Decaffeinated tea and coffee are definitely not the answer, as they will still encourage larger amounts of acid. Read the section on coffee and discover how decaffeinated coffee can be even more acid forming than regular coffee due to the type of coffee bean used.

Foods that heal ulcers are rich in vitamin A, B and C. Cabbage contains vitamin U, known to help ulcers. Carrots, pumpkin, sweet potatoes (yams) are rich in beta-carotene, a precursor to vitamin A, essential to the health of the mucus lining. Vitamin C is important, but you must avoid citrus fruits like oranges, tangerines, etc. Try different fruits to see how they affect you. If fruits cause problems, vegetables are also a good source of vitamin C.

If you think you have a problem - pain after eating, passing very dark or very light stools - visit your doctor, to rule out a bacterial infection or other conditions.

Crohn's Disease

This condition can affect the small or large intestine. The lining of the intestine is very inflamed and ulcerated. Symptoms range from weight loss, many bouts of diarrhea, swollen stomach and fatigue. The loose stools can be mixed with mucus and blood or, in severe cases, pus. There will be stomach bloating, aching muscles, skin rashes and fatigue, often due to nutritional deficiency mainly attributed to malabsorption.

Other common symptoms are fever, anemia and weight loss. In any case of unexplained weight loss (even if the rest of your symptoms are very mild) you should get some tests done. In other words, if you are eating your usual diet without extra physical activity but are losing weight, get checked out by your doctor or naturopathic practitioner.

During an acute phase, a fast is recommended, but only under supervision. It's very important you don't treat Crohn's disease yourself. This condition is in a different league to IBS or piles. However, there is much you can do to improve your situation by changing your diet. First and foremost, remove lactose from your diet - this means all milk and cheese. Try some goat's yogurt, very easy to find in the supermarkets these days. You will also need to eliminate wheat and rye from your diet as well as all sugar, soft drinks, tea and coffee. See also the section on ulcerative colitis.

Ulcerative Colitis

This is a painful condition of the large intestine or colon. Symptoms are blood- and mucus-filled stools, as the ulcers erupt. It can be normal to be in remission for some time and then suddenly get an attack. The main symptoms are poor digestion, weight loss, anemia and diarrhea. The stools can be soft or watery with a sudden urgency to go. For some people, venturing from home can be a problem, as there is a fear that they will not find a toilet in time.

A poor diet over several years would have contributed to this and many other digestive problems. Stress also contributes and will make your symptoms worse. There is a connection between food intolerances and many conditions, especially colitis, and it would certainly be worthwhile finding out what you might have an intolerance to. Check out BANT (British Association of Nutritional Therapy) and ION (Institute of Optimum Nutrition), as they can recommend qualified practitioners in your area, who could advise on food intolerances. Do this after you have seen your doctor and had the necessary tests.

In the case of colitis, you should see your doctor and a qualified nutritional therapist or naturopath, plus you need to take a long hard look at some aspects of your life. Those aspects that are causing too much stress and unhappiness, once identified, should be seriously addressed.

If you have any of these conditions, check out the section on herbs and spices and look up those for improving digestion. You will be able to choose one that suits your symptoms by looking up their individual properties.

Chapter 3

Toxins

"Lunch Hollywood style - a hot dog and vintage wine"
Harry Kurnitz: The Wit and Wisdom of Hollywood

As we all know, toxins are harmful to our bodies. So where do they come from, and how can we avoid them or deal with them?

There are those from our external world and those that are produced in, and come from, our internal world. External toxins include heavy metals such as aluminum, arsenic, cadmium, lead, mercury and nickel. These metals can impair the function of the kidneys, immune system, liver and brain. There are preservatives, artificial sweeteners, colorings, food additives, pesticides, and there are also chemicals from cosmetics, toiletries, pharmaceutical drugs, synthetic vitamins and minerals. And let's not forget the air-borne toxins - emissions from cars, factories, etc.

Internal toxins, produced daily, are normal metabolic by-products.

Toxins need to be dealt with on a daily basis, regardless of their origin. This process puts a heavy demand on our organs of elimination, like the liver, kidneys, bowels, skin and lungs. Most of us make detoxification very difficult for these organs, hindering the process on a daily basis, as opposed to aiding and abetting it.

We become tired, sluggish and a little irritable, we get general aches and pains and headaches. We are led to believe this is normal. If you feel like this, it's time to take a long hard look at your lifestyle (diet and habits) before your symptoms become more serious.

When the body's self-healing, self-cleansing processes become overwhelmed, the immune system can become stressed, leading to chronic degeneration, so common today. We need to give our bodies every opportunity to regenerate and strengthen our immune system.

As toxins build up in our bodies, increasing stress builds up in our organs. When you have a pain like a headache, or frequent infections or digestive complaints, your body is trying to tell you something. Most of us respond by taking painkillers, antibiotics, cholesterol-lowering tablets, diuretics, or antacids. These measures, however, don't solve the problem; they only turn off the body's alarm bells. If your house alarm is set off, do you simply turn off the power supply to stop the noise, or do you find out what set it off in the first place?

When we take a pharmaceutical drug, we suppress our natural healing processes; we turn off the signals, the symptoms. If you are producing too much acid, you need to find out why. Taking an antacid

> *Caffeine*
> *Children are more prone to caffeine's negative effects, yet cola drinks legally contain substantial amounts. A typical cup of coffee contains 90 to 100mg of caffeine. Unfortunately its effects wear off, and very soon we need another cup of coffee or tea or coke or even chocolate. Symptoms generated by this yo-yo effect can include irritability, restlessness, nausea, headaches, tiredness or hyperactivity. This puts unnecessary strain on some of our organs.*
> *Researchers have now come to the conclusion that, if you are pregnant, you need to cut down on your coffee consumption. If you have a history of miscarriages, you need to give up coffee altogether.*

isn't sorting out the cause and, in the long term, could make things worse. I have to say at this point, pharmaceutical drugs, when used correctly, are lifesavers, miracles of science. However, they should be considered after all other avenues have been explored first.

We all lead stressful lives with our careers, families, financial pressures, and around all of that, we try to fit in the gym and a social life. Then, to add insult to injury, we add more stress to our bodies by way of the food and drink we choose to consume. Even the way we eat and drink adds stress. We need to give our bodies the best tools and materials to enable them to detoxify on a daily basis, to stop the process of degeneration and turn it into regeneration. The main aim of detoxification is to encourage the cells to excrete wastes efficiently every day, and for fully functioning organs to handle this waste.

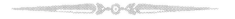

Chapter 4

Vitamins and Minerals

"There is no danger of my getting scurvy, as I have to consume at least two gin-and-limes every evening to keep out the cold"
S.J. Perelman

Vitamins

In order for enzymes to work in the body they need vitamins and minerals, known as co-enzymes. Our bodies need to obtain these co-enzymes from our food, as we are unable to make most of them for ourselves. As we have already discussed, the foods we generally eat are deficient in both enzymes and co-enzymes. For instance, white flour, most people's staple, has had most of the B Vitamins removed. B Vitamins are extremely important co-enzymes, involved in the production of energy. Generally, twenty-two nutrients are removed from flour in the refining process and four or five are replaced, but in a synthetic version. These are added back in some countries by law.

Vitamins are known as micronutrients, as they are required in such small amounts. They are essential molecules necessary for numerous bodily functions. Vitamins are divided into two groups: fat-soluble vitamins and water-soluble vitamins. Vitamins A, D, E, F and K are fat-soluble vitamins, as they need adequate amounts of fat (the correct type) and minerals in the diet for correct absorption. These fat-soluble vitamins are stored in the liver. The body excretes these via the large intestine in our feces. Vitamin C, Bs and P are water-soluble and cannot be stored in the body. These vitamins are absorbed from our intestines and are found bound to enzymes, and any excesses are excreted via the kidneys in urine. The water-soluble vitamins are also essential to our enzyme activity.

No vitamin or mineral acts by itself; it needs to interact with other vitamins and minerals before it can be utilized. For instance, Vitamin C isn't a cure for the common cold, but it is the principal nutrient in raising the body's resistance to the cold and flu virus. The white blood cells cannot absorb Vitamin C unless Vitamins B12 and B6, folic acid, choline and the mineral zinc are present in adequate amounts. This is dependent on the person eating nutritious foods and being able to digest and absorb them properly. I am going to mention each vitamin only briefly, because there are a number of very good books that explain each nutrient in much more depth.

Vitamin A (Retinol) is a fat-soluble antioxidant nutrient that protects the body's cells against attack and builds up resistance to infection. It's essential to the health of the skin and mucous passages (the GI tract as well as the respiratory tract) and for good night-vision. There is another form called beta-carotene found in red, yellow and orange fruit and vegetables. The liver will convert beta-carotene into Vitamin A. Good sources of Vitamin A are animal products.

The B vitamins are needed for the release of energy from our food and for the health of the nervous system and digestive system. These are water-soluble vitamins that are not stored by the body, so they must be obtained from our food on a daily basis. The following vitamins tend to appear together in food:

B1 - thiamine
B2 - riboflavin
B3 - niacin
B5 - pantothenic acid
B6 - pyridoxine
B9 - folic acid
B12 - cobalamin
Biotin
Choline
Inositol

B Vitamins tend to appear together in food. Most are lost in the processing of food, especially white rice and white flour. Those who are drinkers or smokers, or those who use the contraceptive pill or HRT (hormone replacement therapy), or those who are under a lot of stress or rely on junk and processed foods will have an increased need for B Vitamins. If you want to take any B Vitamins, then always take these as a 'B complex', unless otherwise prescribed by a practitioner. B Vitamins are found in whole grains, lentils, eggs and green vegetables.

Choline is sometimes classified as a B Vitamin, but there is some dispute about this fact. We get a considerable amount from our diet, and we can also synthesize it, given the right raw materials. Choline is particularly concerned with nerve transmission and with the maintenance of cell membranes. It's especially important to the brain function. The richest sources come from egg yolks, whole grains, legumes (beans and lentils), peanuts and liver.

Vitamin C (ascorbic acid) is essential to the health of the skin, hair, gums, bones and ligaments. Its main function is the repair and growth of the body tissue and the maintenance of healthy blood vessels and red blood cells, fighting off free radicals and keeping the immune system in good order. It aids in the absorption of iron. Most animals produce their own Vitamin C, but we need a daily supply from our food. It's a water-soluble vitamin that cannot be stored in the body. It's very unstable in fresh food and it can easily be destroyed by oxygen, light and heat. Buy fresh fruit and vegetables, store them in the fridge and use them as soon as possible. Steam vegetables lightly or eat them raw.

Vitamin D is called the 'sunshine' vitamin, as it's formed in the skin and activated by the sun. Vitamin D enables the body to utilize calcium and phosphorus, encouraging strong teeth and bones. Vitamin D can be stored in the body, so never take more than the recommended dose. Calciperol is the synthetically produced Vitamin D.

Vitamin E is a fat-soluble vitamin. It's a powerful antioxidant, protecting or delaying the onset of diseases associated with ageing. Vitamin E helps maintain a healthy circulation by keeping the blood vessel walls clear and healthy. Nuts and seeds are a good source - although it's very important not to eat roasted ones. Natural supplements are labeled d-alpha tocopherol, synthetic ones are labeled dl-alpha tocopherol. In studies, the natural Vitamin E was found to be one-third more potent, and twice as effective as the synthetic version.

Vitamin K is a fat-soluble vitamin that plays an essential role in normal blood clotting and liver function. This isn't available as a supplement on its own, but it can be found in some multi vitamin/mineral formulas. A good source is dark green leafy vegetables, alfalfa sprouts and mustard greens.

Vitamin P is known as a bioflavonoid. This is a group of phyto-nutrients that are found with Vitamin C in all fruit and vegetables. Each encourages the absorption of the other.

One can find *Vitamin U* in cabbage. Scientists named this compound Vitamin U because it was found to help heal ulcers.

Slow-Release Vitamins

Some supplements are labeled 'slow-release', 'time release' or 'sustained release'. They claim to release their ingredients into the body over a period of time. Absorption of any nutrient depends on the way in which it's digested, in addition to the dose. There has always been a question mark over this type of supplement and its claim. The water-soluble vitamins like B and C can be presented in this way. These products are presented as capsules containing tiny 'beads' of nutrients or as specially coated tablets, which slowly erode as they pass through the digestive process. They tend to be more expensive.

Minerals

Minerals are also known as micro minerals or trace elements, performing many roles within the body. Minerals that the body needs in larger quantities are calcium, phosphate, potassium and magnesium. Minerals needed in smaller amounts are iron, zinc, chromium, manganese, copper, iodine, selenium, fluoride, molybdenum and cobalt. Minerals originate from the soil and are taken up by the plants, then utilized by us because the plants have converted them into a form that is bio-available to us. The same goes for farm animals that eat the plants, because they provide us with minerals in a form we can readily absorb. Many minerals are lost in food processing and refining.

For instance, zinc is needed to help make the correct formation of hydrochloric acid, which will aid the proper functioning of our taste buds. A shortage of zinc can cause our food to taste bland and this encourages us to add too much salt to our food in compensation. This can cause further health problems, and salt also inhibits our enzyme activity. Zinc assists many enzymes to metabolize carbohydrates. Zinc helps to fight infections and speeds up healing of wounds, and it also affects thyroid function, works with insulin, even helps to protect against heavy metal poisoning. Most of us don't get enough minerals.

Vitamins and minerals are both measured in milligrams (mg). A milligram is a thousandth of a gram. They can also be measured in micrograms (mcg). A microgram is a millionth of a gram. Vitamin E is measured in international units (iu), and one gram equals 1.5iu.

Boron is a trace mineral found in most plants. It's essential for healthy bones and muscles. Research shows that boron slows down the loss of calcium and magnesium from the bones.

Calcium, as we all know, is needed for the bones, teeth, nerves, muscles and blood. Calcium promotes sleep, and keeps the heart beating and the muscles contracting. If you decide to take calcium, make sure you take it with other nutrients that aid its absorption. Good sources are yogurts, almonds and sesame seeds, and also dark-green leafy vegetables.

Chromium is a trace mineral involved in the metabolism and in particular with the production of insulin. Chromium lowers cholesterol and other fats in the blood. Molasses are a good source.

Copper is required in respiration to convert iron into hemoglobin. Copper utilizes the amino acid tyrosine, allowing it to work as a pigment for hair and skin.

Iodine is a trace element that is essential for the formation of thyroxin and tri-iodothyroxin. An iodine deficiency can lead to an under active thyroid, with symptoms such as lack of energy, weight gain, dry skin, feeling cold and slowing down of all body functions. Before you start to panic, some of the above symptoms could be related to many different conditions including lack of sleep, stress or lack of other nutrients, etc. Seaweeds are a good source of iodine.

Iron is a metal that is used by the body to make hemoglobin. This is the red pigment in blood. Hemoglobin carries oxygen around the body. Good food sources are dark-green vegetables and meat.

Magnesium is a vital component of bones and teeth. It's closely involved in the release of energy and the correct functioning of the nerves and muscles. Good sources are fish, beans, nuts, seeds and green vegetables.

Manganese is essential to the function of the pituitary gland, the brain, and nerve and muscle action throughout the body. It is vital to the body's antioxidant defense system. The body needs manganese to make interferon, a natural anti-viral agent. Sources are oats, nuts, buckwheat, green tea, and whole grains.

Molybdenum is essential for reproductive health and it helps the body to detoxify and rid itself of chemical additives. It's found in whole grains, beans and lentils, leafy green vegetables and goat's milk.

Phosphorus is present in every cell in the body, and it's involved in most of the body's physiological chemical reactions. It's needed for strong bones and teeth. This mineral is never taken as a supplement on its own.

Potassium controls the acid/alkaline balance. It's found in fruit and vegetables and it works with other nutrients to form essential electrically charged ions known as electrolytes that make up the fluids in the body. Potassium is crucial to many functions, including the heartbeat, energy production, nerve conduction, blood pressure, and muscle contraction.

Selenium is an important antioxidant that works in conjunction with Vitamin E. Selenium boosts the immune system, keeps the liver healthy and combats the ageing process. Selenium is present in fish and whole grains.

Silicon (is also known as silica) is the most plentiful element after oxygen. Chemical fertilizers and food processing tend to deplete it. In the body, silicon is a vital part of connective tissue, bones, blood vessels and cartilage. It helps strengthen the skin, hair and nails by improving the production of collagen and keratin, the proteins found in the joints, hair and nails. Good sources are oats, barley and brown rice.

Sulfur keeps skin and hair healthy. Eggs, onions and garlic provide sulfur.

Vanadium is believed to inhibit the formation of cholesterol in the blood vessels, and this mineral appears in tiny amounts in many foods. Good sources are black pepper, dill seeds, aniseed, celery seed and fenugreek seeds.

Zinc is essential to over eighty processes and enzymes. It helps to maintain a healthy immune system, it's involved in repairing damaged tissue, it helps to maintain a healthy sperm count and it aids the ability to taste and smell properly. Zinc is found in whole grains and some nuts and seeds, especially pumpkin seeds.

Chelation (pronounced key-la-tion) is a process by which mineral supplements are made more absorbable. For example, the label on the supplement container might state magnesium as 'amino acid chelated'.

Where do these important enzymes and co-enzymes come from? In theory, this is easy to answer, but in practice, not so easy. They come from fresh fruit and vegetables, from raw nuts and seeds, yogurt, legumes and whole grains. Few people eat these sorts of foods on a regular basis.

Most of us don't get enough enzymes and co-enzymes. Consider how you live and the fresh foods that you eat on a daily basis. Keeping a daily food and drink diary will give you a very clear picture. Many people tell me, when they look back over records that they have kept for a week or two, how totally surprised they are. Most of us only really get the full picture when we see it in black and white. A food diary is well worth the effort.

Increasing Your Co-Enzyme Intake
Here are a few foods that will help you to achieve this:
Natural live yogurt
Sprouted beans, seeds, grains, lentils, etc
Juiced fruit and vegetables
Lightly steamed vegetables
Grains soaked overnight - for instance, muesli
Raw nuts, seeds, fruit and vegetables

Sauerkraut is salted cabbage. This helps to enhance absorption and encourages a healthful intestinal flora. It's very salty, but it isn't something that anyone eats a great deal of at any one time, so the high salt content doesn't matter too much. Captain Cook insisted that his crew ate a little sauerkraut every day while on their voyages. This prevented the men from developing scurvy and other ailments that come from going a long time with no fresh fruit and vegetables and thus depriving them of Vitamin C, among other things. The crew soon grew to hate the sauerkraut but they preferred eating it to getting a few dozen lashes for insubordination!

Miso is a fermented soybean, barley or rice paste. It's fermented for six months to two years. There are many types, with their own distinctive flavors. It's a 'live' food that contains lactobacillus (like yogurt), so one should use this instead of stock cubes. This sounds dreadful to our western minds, but having eaten miso soup in the Far East and also in Japanese restaurants in England, I can give you the surprising news that it tastes very nice indeed.

Coenzyme Q10 is found in every cell in the body. It's essential for generating energy in all living things that use oxygen. Coenzyme Q10 is found in all fresh food, but is easily destroyed by cooking. It's an antioxidant, and has been found to be as powerful as Vitamin E. The highest concentrations are found in the heart, then the liver and the immune system. It's a good reason for including some fresh raw foods in our daily diets.

Temperature

At approximately 60°C, which is about 140°F, enzymes are destroyed. Pasteurization is a method of using high temperatures (especially for milk) that destroys all the enzymes. This process is also used in other industries, not just the dairy industry, so you may find that fruit juices have been treated in this way. The canning industry also uses high temperatures, thus killing enzyme activity. In this process, most nutrients are lost or destroyed.

Frozen vegetables are better than canned vegetables, but they are never as good as fresh vegetables. Before vegetables are frozen, they are first blanched. This inhibits enzyme activity and causes water-soluble vitamins to be washed away. Sun-dried food has also had some of its enzymes destroyed. You may well be eating plenty of vegetables, but you can destroy enzymes by the way you cook and store them. Most people boil their vegetables for too long in water, destroying enzymes. Then they throw valuable nutrients down the drain, literally!

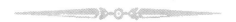

Chapter 5

Antioxidants

"Never serve oysters in a month that has no paycheck in it"
P. J. O'Rourke: The Bachelor Home Companion

I am sure we have all heard of antioxidants and free radicals. Firstly, free radicals attack us in a similar way that an iron gate can end up rusty if not adequately protected. Cut open an apple and watch the cut surface go brown - it's the oxygen. Free radicals attack us on a daily basis, causing anything from wrinkles to cancer. You paint your iron gate to protect it from rusting. In the same way, we can protect and slow down the damage of free radicals by consuming antioxidants - zinc, selenium, Vitamins C, E, and A. There are also phyto-nutrients or phyto-chemicals, known as plant compounds. These antioxidants are like anti-rust compounds.

Some of the worst causes of free radical damage are smoking cigarettes, too much exposure to UVs from the sun, damaged fats (more on this subject later), and pollutants like exhaust fumes. Nature has provided foods that are rich in antioxidants, as well as enzymes and co-enzymes, namely fresh fruit and vegetables.

Here is a very small list taken from the hundreds of plant compounds that have powerful healing, protective and detoxification properties. They are anti-inflammatory and anti-cancerous, helping to lower blood pressure, prevent blood clots, strengthen the capillaries and much more.

Quercetin is one of the bioflavonoids, with anti-inflammatory, anti-oxidant and anti-histamine properties. Quercetin may also help prevent or slow down nerve, eye, and kidney damage for those with diabetes. Found in onions.

Rutin is an antioxidative vitamin-like substance from the bioflavonoid group. Rutin supplements are used in the treatment of capillary fragility and bruising - typical of many people with high blood pressure - as well as bleeding gums. Buckwheat is a good source of rutin.

Ellagic acid, a phyto-chemical found in cherries, grapes and strawberries, protects against cancer and other degenerative diseases.

Cruciferous indoles, found in vegetables like broccoli, cabbage, and Brussels sprouts, protect against cancer and other degenerative diseases.

Genistein is a phyto-chemical derived from soya beans, high in isoflavones, which normalizes the activity of estrogen/testosterone.

Glucarates are found in lemons, grapefruits and whole grains, improving detoxification.

Lignins are found in linseeds, carrots, beans, peas, whole grains and some fruits; they lower cholesterol, normalizing the metabolism of testosterone/testosterone.

Saponins, found in legumes (beans and lentils), have anticancer properties.

Carotenoids are found in orange and yellow colored fruit and vegetables like apricots, pumpkins, carrots etc., and aid in the protection of Vitamin A.

Our Life Span

According to some studies, our life span should be at least 100 to 110 years! This may surprise you. Certain criteria have been established that are important to quality and quantity of life.

We need to maintain:
~   An even weight that is normal for us; no yo-yo weight gain and loss.
~   Good nutrition - health enhancing foods and supplements.
~   A positive outlook.

These days, it's impossible to avoid all pollutants and toxins. We can, however, minimize the damage they cause us. Each and every one of our cells has its own predetermined life span. Some have hours to live, others days or months. Most cells are no longer able to reproduce correct copies of themselves after they have divided about fifty times. Under normal circumstances, they self-destruct.

Research has revealed that the rate at which we age is genetically predetermined. So why bother, why worry? Let's just go out and party; we are going to die at a given time, anyway. Well, the choice is simple, you can enhance your situation and try to reach your full potential, or continue as you are, and accelerate the degeneration. We all have to make the most of what we have been given. If our genes have predetermined that we live until our mid seventies or mid nineties, let us try and make sure we do everything possible to make them healthy, active, pain free, and happy years.

It has been shown that as we age, our immune system becomes weaker, making us more susceptible to infections. I know what you are thinking. We are often told that, according to statistics, we are living longer these days, despite our Western diet. In our recent history, the child mortality rate was very high. Most families would have suffered the loss of a baby or a child, as this was commonplace. It would have been rare to hear of a family that had not been touched in this way. Today, the opposite is true: we rarely meet families who have lost children. This fact would have had a very big impact on the average age calculated, bringing the age down. And, of course, medicine has added quantity to our lives, though not always quality.

However, our aim here should be to add quality to our lives, not just quantity. As I said earlier, ageing is inevitable, but so much chronic suffering is not.

Quality Of Life

We all want to feel better, look better and live a longer life. I don't have aspirations to live to be 100 or 110. However, if I am going to live to eighty-eight, for instance, then at least I want those later years to be productive and fulfilling.

If we consider anything that is worth having, then it's usually something we have to work for. Those qualifications need to be revised for, that medal needs to be trained for, or that award needs to be practiced for. Few of us have a natural gift. Where health is concerned, few of us can eat junk, smoke and drink too much, and still live an energetic, pain-free life. Most of us would like to think we could eat and drink what we like and then pop a multi-vitamin and mineral, or an antacid, and still expect to stay energetic and looking good.

In truth, we all want an easy life, an easy quick fix. A 'quick fix', if there were such a thing, would leave us all fit and feeling great. However, in truth, most of us have to work at staying healthy.

Those of you who are prepared to make a few changes to your lifestyle will reap huge benefits in both the short term and the long term. This book will help you to achieve these benefits in a simple, achievable way. There are no agonizing exercises, no starvation regime, no strange rituals, no drugs, and no expensive concoctions.

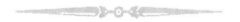

Chapter 6

Acid/Alkaline Balance

"Food that to him now is as luscious as locusts,
shall be to him shortly as bitter as coloquintida
Ibid, 354

Under normal circumstances our blood should be slightly alkaline, ensuring cells are well oxygenated. When we bombard our bodies with more toxins than it can handle, we become more acidic and oxygen levels to the cells drop. This situation sets up the perfect environment for bacteria, viruses and fungus infections to thrive. A toxic condition provides the perfect breeding ground for germs.

We are led to believe that most illnesses are genetic and that there is little we can do about them. I find this a strange statement; if this is the case, why are most chronic diseases many times more prevalent today? If we look at every situation where native people changed from a 'traditional diet' to a Western-type diet, they have begun to suffer diseases that were rare in their traditional societies but common in our societies.

This isn't genetic inheritance, but it is adopting our eating habits, inheriting our way of life and hence our chronic diseases. There is also a vast amount of research exposing the fact that there is much we can do to prevent cancer, and that our present lifestyles are enhancing our chances of developing certain types of cancer.

Back in 1931, Dr Otto Warbury received the Nobel Prize for Medicine for his work on cancer. His discovery was that all forms of cancer like to thrive in an environment that is acidic and lacks oxygen - acidosis and hypoxia. Many researchers have verified this since: cancer cells love an anaerobic (lack of oxygen) environment where they can reproduce fast. It's important to all aspects of our health that we encourage an alkaline environment, where cells are well oxygenated.

Flushing out Acidity

Almost all toxins cause acidity. Every cell in the body is reliant on blood for its supply of vital nutrients, and for it to remove waste from metabolism and from the breakdown of worn-out parts. Slightly acidic, polluted blood will not be able to keep our cells well stocked and cleansed. The lymph, if congested, will also do a poor job. The lymph, unlike the blood stream, does not have a pump (the heart) ensuring its flow around our body. The lymph has to rely on muscles and physical movement. The more active we are, the better our lymph will flow. Acidity will interfere with an already vulnerable system as many of us lead very sedentary lives. The blood and lymph systems are like the drainage systems of our homes, they need to be kept clean and unblocked, at all times. Our drainage system needs to be continually flushed out with cleansing fluids.

However, too many people are dehydrated. Most people drink too much tea, coffee and soft drinks, which are acid forming and encourage the kidneys to excrete more fluid, encouraging dehydration. We just don't drink enough hydrating fluids. In my practice I come across a lot of people who say to me, 'I don't like water', 'I can't drink water because it makes me feel sick', or 'I don't like cold drinks'. I will explain a little later how we can get around these problems.

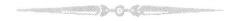

Chapter 7

Water

"Water is the only drink for a wise man"
Henry David Thoreau, nineteenth-century ecologist.

The human body is made up mostly of water. All the chemical reactions needed to produce heat and energy, that enable us to think, feel, emote, express, see, hear and move take place in this water.

Falling levels of water pressure in the blood vessels, due to dehydration, will mean fewer nutrients like oxygen, vitamins, minerals and proteins are being forced into the cells. The cells rely on this fluid to carry nutrients in and flush their waste products out. If the waste products lie around in the cell, they interfere with normal chemical reactions, and so unbalance the metabolism. When the osmotic pulling power of the blood is reduced, fewer waste products are drawn out from the cells into to the blood for elimination through the kidneys, and the more acidic the environment becomes.

Water doesn't need explaining, nor do I need to tell you how important it is. Or do I? Survey after survey, case study after case study tells a different story. We are not taking water seriously enough. Research reveals that most of us are dehydrated and that some of us are very dehydrated, causing long-term health problems. Being dehydrated is more serious than you would think.

Water is the second most important nutrient, after oxygen. Our brains are made up of nearly eighty-five per cent water, and solid tissue, like muscle, which is made up of about seventy per cent water. A lot of people including children are drinking themselves into dehydration by consuming too little water and too many beverages that rob our body of fluids. Most of us are probably only getting about a third of the valuable hydration benefits we need.

Water is important in nearly every major function in the body. It's a major component of blood and contains much dissolved oxygen that is easily assimilated into the body, it helps prevent constipation, and it flushes the body of metabolic wastes. Water helps maintain muscle tone (a dehydrated muscle is a stiff muscle and more likely to injure). It acts like a natural 'air conditioner', regulating body temperature. It's crucial for metabolic reactions: when the body becomes dehydrated metabolism slows down, leading to a substantial decrease in energy.

The six to eight glasses we are recommended to drink each day is only a general guide line, as much will depend on your body size, your level of activity, how much dehydrating food and drink you consume, how much stress you have to cope with and how hot it is. Unfortunately, people under a lot of stress reach for more coffee or tea or alcohol, which are all dehydrating, causing more stress under an already stressful situation.

Water is needed for the breakdown of protein, so if you increase your protein intake (as with some popular high-protein slimming programs), your consumption of water should also be increased. If you smoke or drink alcohol regularly, water is crucial for removing metabolic waste from the body. In fact, water is called the universal solvent, since it's capable of dissolving and carrying nearly any kind of matter, including toxins.

Improving Your Water's Purity

Water is the indispensable inorganic element that dissolves, transports, lubricates, purifies, moistens and generally keeps us alive. The researchers at the School of Public Health at the University of California estimate that several million complex bio-molecules are now present in various water supplies. One particularly disturbing example is the case of chlorine. Greenpeace have stated that forty million tons of chlorine are used by industry worldwide each year. Chlorinated compounds have been detected in the polar icecap, and 177 organochlorines have been detected in humans!

Another serious area of concern is pollution from estrogens and chemicals that mimic estrogens. These come from birth control pills, hormone replacement therapy and other sources. Research by John Sumper, Professor of Biology at Brunel University, has studied the phenomenon of feminized male fish living in water found to contain estrogenic substances. As estrogenic chemicals of various kinds are accumulating in the environment, it may be wiser to take steps to remove oestrogens from drinking water, rather than wait for research to confirm the same fate for human males!

The healthful state of our body cells is maintained by the constant process of renewal, provided the cells can be replaced according to the original 'memory' or blueprint. Anything that interferes with this copying process will contribute to ageing. The more complicated the pollutants in our cooking and drinking water, the more difficult the process of cleansing, cell renewal and nutrient transport becomes.

The following information is about the most commonly used methods for improving the quality of our drinking water. The various methods of filtration and purification aim to remove three types of contamination: Biological - bacteria, viruses, helminths (worms), and protozoa (parasites); chemical - pesticides, herbicides, solvents, chlorine, organochlorines, and hundreds of other chemicals, and aesthelic - dust, silt, rust, sand, etc.

Reverse osmosis is a technique of forcing water, by electric pump or mains pressure, through a semi-permeable membrane. This synthetic membrane is a chemical compound, which has relative stability. Some RO units allow volatile organic chemicals to pass through. This is the reason some units include an activated carbon filter. RO has the ability to remove salt and so is often used for the desalination of seawater. RO also removes naturally occurring minerals and so has a softening effect on water.

Granulated activated carbon is found in the most widely used filters including jugs, tap-mounted and most under-sink units. The main filtering effect is achieved by water passing slowly through the carbon granules, which have an enormous total surface area. This functions as an electro-chemical absorbent sieve, removing various contaminants including chlorine, hence the improved taste and appearance. To prevent the build-up of bacteria inside the cartridge, the carbon granules have been impregnated with silver.

Ceramic filtration is a technique that has been used for years. The effectiveness of ceramics depends on their pore size; the smallest goes down to one micron. Plenty of known chemicals and bacteria can pass through. This type of filter can be a good starting point for multi-stage filtration.

Multi-stage or combination filters are devices that use a combination of methods that can greatly improve the quality of drinking water. This is the sophisticated end of the filter market. Such a product can give up to ninety-three per cent removal of contaminants across a wide range of biological and chemical offenders. Naturally occurring minerals are not removed.

A submicron matrix purifier is an advanced system allowing filtration down to 0.1 micron. Particles within the matrix have positive and negative charges. Certain disease-causing bacteria are as small as 0.5 microns. This system doesn't remove naturally occurring minerals. Published research indicates 97 to 99.9 per cent purification throughout the life of each cartridge. Variations in design include under-sink, counter-top, portable or large-volume units.

When considering which unit or system to buy, more important than the initial purchase cost is the ongoing cost. Some of the more expensive units do a better job and their running costs can be a lot lower.

Bottled Water

Factors we need to consider when buying water are the cost, the amount of plastic or glass used in the manufacturing process, disposal or recycling of bottles, and the overall environmental impact including transportation. Surveys have revealed bacteria in some bottled water, although not always unfriendly. Also, sometimes minerals levels of nitrates can be too high for very young children.

Club soda is also artificially carbonated filtered water, but contains added minerals salts.

Demineralized water has been neutralized by the addition or removal of electrons, and the resulting water is called de-ionized or de-mineralized. This process removes nitrates and the minerals calcium and magnesium, plus the heavy metals cadmium, barium, lead and some forms of radium.

Mineral water is natural spring water, usually from Europe or Canada. To be considered mineral water, in addition to containing minerals, the water must flow freely from its source, it cannot be pumped or forced from the ground in any way, and must be bottled at source.

Natural spring water. The word 'natural' on the label does not tell you where the water comes from; only that the mineral content has not been altered. It may even be possible that the water didn't come from a spring.

Spring water, generally, is water that rises naturally to the earth's surface from underground reservoirs. The water is unprocessed, though flavor or carbonation may be added.

Sparkling water is water that has been carbonated.

'Naturally sparkling water' must get its carbonation from the same source as the water.

'Carbonated natural water' means the carbonation has come from a source other than the one that supplied the water. This does not mean the quality of this water is poor, as its mineral content is still the same as when it came out of the ground.

Carbonated fluids can be irritating to the gastrointestinal tract.

Steamed-distilled water means vaporizing the water by boiling it. The steam rises, leaving behind bacteria, chemicals, minerals and any pollutants. Once in the body, steam-distilled water will remove minerals and toxins rejected by the cells and tissues.

Fluid Loss

We lose almost a liter (two pints) of fluid through our lungs and skin just in breathing each day! Yes, our skin does breath. Of course this amount can rise, if the weather is hot, if we work physically hard or train a lot.

pH Balance

We need to restore the correct pH balance to our blood on a daily basis.

---

pH Levels:
1 = extremely acidic
7 = neutral
14 = extremely alkaline

Our blood should be 7.3 to 7.4

So, what are some of the consequences of slightly too much acidity in the blood and other systems that should normally be slightly on the alkaline side?

1. The heart pumps about 130 liters of blood per hour. Amazing when you think about all that activity going unnoticed.
2. Normal heartbeat is dependent on slightly alkaline blood.
3. Acidic levels will eventually cause deterioration to the heart tissue.
4. Too much acidic waste in the blood will seriously reduce its oxygen-carrying capacity, having a negative affect on every cell in our body.

Dehydration

You seriously need to think about your fluid intake. I come across a lot of tired people. There are many reasons for fatigue but one of the main reasons is dehydration.

Research has revealed that people who drink five to eight glasses of water a day reduced their risk of all sorts of cancers and other diseases. Drinking this amount of water also relieved pain and joint stiffness. If you suffer from headaches, maybe you are not drinking enough hydrating fluids. When you are dehydrated your cells contract and retain waste. When you are well hydrated your cells expand, allowing them to get rid of their waste products, and to maintain the correct pH balance.

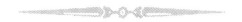

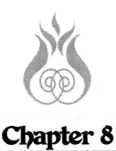

Chapter 8

Major Organs of Elimination

"Weak food best fits weak stomachs"
15th century proverb

There are five major routes of elimination, hence five major organs working day and night trying to maintain equilibrium by removing waste every minute of the day. They are hard-working organs that all work together, but can easily be overwhelmed by the choices we make every day.

Lungs

Breathing is an important way for the body to regulate the body's pH levels. Breathing well saturates the blood with fresh oxygen, and at the same time gets rid of carbon dioxide. Oxygen supports an alkaline environment in the blood and tissues. On the other hand, carbon dioxide encourages an acid environment.

Liver

One of its major roles is to filter out toxins from the bloodstream. The blood is constantly being bombarded with pollutants, from one source or another. They can come from what we eat and drink, plus some of the social habits we have developed, like too much alcohol, smoking or being dependent on painkillers, or taking 'the pill', for instance. If you have decided that taking 'the pill' is your only sensible option for contraception, then just make sure you balance your decision with a good diet and some basic supplements. If you smoke, try giving up.

The liver produces many alkaline-forming enzymes. It breaks down chemicals and pharmaceutical drugs to less harmful substances ready for disposal. In this age of more air pollutants, more pollutants in our drinking water, more chemicals being sprayed on our foods, more food additives and preservatives, we are giving our livers far too much to do, often without all the necessary tools and materials to do its job.

> *To help the liver, squeeze the juice of half a fresh lemon into*
> *a little warm water and drink it first thing in the morning.*
> *Taking lecithin granules will also help the liver.*
> *Making some of the diet changes suggested in this book will help*
> *the liver enormously.*

Skin

The skin is a huge detoxifying organ. I should think you have never thought of your skin as an organ. It accounts for about sixteen per cent of our body weight. It's shed and renewed at a rate of about 1oz or 25g every month. The skin excretes an enormous amount of toxic waste each day, especially in the summer, as the pores remain open. In the winter saunas and steam baths will open up the pores and encourage cleansing via the skin.

A well-known and easy way to help the body remove toxins is to soak in a bath of warm/hot water with Epsom salts. Epsom salts can be bought from your local pharmacy or drug store. Ask them to get large packets for you, as this is more economical. If you don't have a bathtub or only like showering, then soak your feet in a bowl of hot water with Epsom salts. This salty water is also very good for draining toxins from the lymph channels and out through the pores of the feet. If you live by the sea, go swimming, providing the water isn't polluted. Unfortunately, most coastal waters are polluted to one degree or another.

Unlike our internal environment, which needs to be slightly alkaline, our external environment needs to be slightly acidic. This helps to protect us from pathogens. While we are on the subject of external environment, our intestines are classed as having an external environment (which may sound a little strange) and hence need to be slightly acid also. Food only enters into our internal environment when it passes through the walls of the intestines, into our blood and lymph and on to our liver.

Harsh soaps can destroy the correct pH levels of the skin. Use mild soaps and shampoos, especially made from plant products. Avoid antiperspirants; use deodorants instead, and look out for the ones that are aluminum-free. Your skin is able to breath better if you wear natural fiber clothes. If you do wear synthetic clothes then try to wear natural fiber underwear. If you wear nightclothes, make sure they are made from natural fibers, and the same goes for your bed covers.

Adding only a little apple cider vinegar to your bath water and to the final rinse after shampooing your hair will help to maintain the correct pH of your skin. If the smell bothers you (it shouldn't do, as the solution is quite dilute), add a couple of drops of essential oil to the water/vinegar mixture.

Kidneys

We have two kidneys, one on either side of the spine, above the waist. They filter 900 liters of blood a day. They are extremely hard-working organs, balancing nutrients and fluid levels, as well as excreting excess sodium, water and end products of metabolism, including heavy metals. The kidneys are constantly dealing with the results of amino acid (protein) breakdown - ammonia and uric acid. When we use fat instead of carbohydrates, as in a 'high-protein diet', ketones are produced. These need to be removed by the kidneys, putting a lot of extra stress on them.

Excess acid waste from a poor diet, pharmaceutical drugs and alcohol can cause the delicate tissues of the filters to become irritated and inflamed and can eventually cause damage.

Most of us are chronically dehydrated and our urine is often more concentrated than it should be. The more concentrated our urine is, the more acidic it will be, which also increases the likelihood of inflammation and irritation, increasing the chance of tissue damage. Water and/or herbal teas are vital in aiding the kidney's very important mission.

Large Intestine (Colon or Bowels)

We need to get our large intestine working better. Generally most of us need to speed up the transition time. If you have had persistent diarrhea, see a naturopath or your doctor. If the transition time is too fast, you may not have time to absorb enough nutrients and fluids, leading to malnutrition and dehydration. For the rest of us, bouts of constipation are more common. Plenty of vegetables and fruit are needed, plus some whole-foods, grains and pulses as they all provide fluids, fiber and cleansing enzymes and nutrients.

These properties encourage the bowels to cleanse, as the transition of waste is speeded up and these foods also encourage 'friendly bacteria', our bowel flora.

Bowel Flora

The average person carries around about three pounds of living bacteria in their intestines. There is an enormous variety and diversity of species, having a negative or positive effect on our whole body. The type of bacteria in our intestines has a huge controlling influence over absorption and our general well being. The environment in our intestines needs to be a little more acidic. This is achieved by cultivating the correct bacteria, known as 'friendly bacteria'. If the environment is too alkaline, the wrong bacteria thrive; the so-called 'unfriendly bacteria' that can cause a large amount of auto-intoxication. Auto-intoxication means our blood stream absorbs toxins produced by our 'unfriendly bacteria'. This creates a huge additional burden for the cleansing abilities of the liver. However, 'friendly bacteria' produce antibodies capable of rendering certain bacteria inactive, contributing to our overall health.

What Encourages the Wrong Bacteria?

A diet with plenty of meat, wheat, sugar, milk and chocolate, tea and coffee does, along with smoking, too much alcohol, antibiotics and steroids (which includes the contraceptive pill), encourage an alkaline environment and hence the 'unfriendly' bacteria.

So what encourages a slightly acidic environment? The answer is, as usual, a diet high in plant-based foods. This includes fruit, vegetables, whole grains, beans, lentils, and products that contain 'friendly bacteria' like yogurt. These 'friendly bacteria' help to produce Vitamins B and K, and aids in their absorption, as well as producing compounds that aid and protect our immune system.

So, a good diet is vital to our long-term health, but is almost wasted if our digestive system isn't working as well as it could, and absorption of nutrients is hindered to a lesser or greater extent.

What Is Our First Priority?

We must prevent constipation or treat diarrhea. If our large bowel isn't functioning properly, we encourage auto-intoxication. If more fluids and toxins are reabsorbed from the bowel back into the bloodstream than is necessary we are putting considerable extra strain on our already overworked liver. Just because you 'go' every day doesn't necessarily mean your intestines are functioning properly or your bowel flora is as it should be.

Fiber

Natural fiber promotes good health in many ways:

1. It provides bulk and holds on to fluid, making our stools softer and therefore much easier to pass.
2. Fiber encourages the correct bacterial balance in our bowels. Fiber is food for the 'friendly bacteria'.
3. Certain types of fiber can help to prevent cancers like breast, prostate and bowel.
4. Certain types of fiber, called soluble, help to lower levels of cholesterol.
5. Fiber also speeds up the transition of waste out of the body. This ensures that auto-intoxication is kept to a minimum.
6. Fiber in natural food helps to keep our blood sugar levels stable.
7. We also feel more satisfied and less likely to overeat, if our diet is full of whole foods, which contain a balance of fiber and nutrients.

Internal Environment

Achieving a more alkaline internal environment is relatively easy. There is no magic, no complicated routines. We just need to include more alkaline-forming foods, while at the same time reducing the amount of acid-forming foods. As we also start to hydrate, we start to give our bodies the tools to flush out toxins, turning degeneration into regeneration. 'Juicing' is just one way; it's extremely effective at flushing out toxins, nourishing the body and balancing our pH levels. We will discuss juicing in more detail later.

Minerals

A good supply of minerals is vital for maintaining acid/alkaline levels. Unfortunately, most people are deficient in many minerals, not getting a good daily supply. If your diet is high in meat, sugar, coffee, dairy products, chocolate and refined wheat, you are maintaining an acid environment that your body is constantly trying to neutralize, and it does this by using alkalizing salts. The main one is calcium, and your body has a huge store it can draw from - your bones and teeth. Our body takes calcium from our bones in an effort to maintain a slightly alkaline balance in the blood, while at the same time we are constantly encouraging slightly acid levels with our dietary habits and addictions. I would like to think of you beginning to act as a friend to your body, not a foe.

Just as it took time for your body to get into a state of degeneration, the reverse is also true; the process of regeneration will also take a little time. Detoxifying should be done slowly and carefully. Better to start off slowly and master it, rather than to start off too fast with too much enthusiasm and then give up. It's like learning to drive, it seems difficult at first, but with time, it becomes so easy it's almost automatic.

Our organs are already working hard, so why would we want to make their job even more difficult, burdening them with more than is necessary?

During detoxification, we encourage our cells to release waste into the bloodstream, where the organs of elimination must cope with the extra load. Stirring up more than these organs can deal with isn't a good idea. We will feel very uncomfortable due to any surplus toxins that cannot always be dealt with, due to an overload, which will only settle back down into the cells again. So, regeneration is taken slowly, allowing our organs to handle the extra without overwhelming them.

We clearly have systems set up for cleansing and regeneration. They are designed to handle waste on a daily basis, within reason. That is the point - within reason. We are overloading our bodies with too many artificial substances and eat too many dead and nutrient-poor foods. We can't expect our bodies to continue like this without eventually suffering the consequences. If you decide to embark on this lifestyle change from degeneration to regeneration, the rewards will be enormous.

Constipation

Constipation is a common complaint. If you are constipated you need to make this your first priority. Solving this problem will have a profound effect on your health. There are several things you can do and naturopathic treatments are always holistic, enhancing the health of the whole body.

Laxatives are not a good idea in the long run. They can cause potassium and fluid loss, leading to further dehydration. A lot of laxatives are irritating, stimulating the nerves to encourage a bowel movement (peristalsis). Eventually, a dependency develops due to muscle weakness, and ultimately causes constipation, the very condition you are trying to solve.

Hydrating Fluids	Dehydrating Fluids
Water	Coffee
Herbal teas	Tea
Fruity teas	Soft drinks
Fruit juice with water	Chocolate drinks
Vegetable juices	Milk shakes
	Alcohol

Here are four steps that will help to solve the problem of constipation:

1. Cut down or give up dehydrating drinks, and add hydrating drinks to your daily routine - see the lists below.
2. Add far more fresh fruit and vegetables to your daily diet.
    I am sure you have noticed that nature has provided us with plenty of watery fruit and vegetables in the summer, such as watermelon and cucumbers. In the more wintry months nature has provided us with more starchy vegetables like pumpkins and parsnips.
    They provide fiber, fluid and nutrients in varying degrees, and all of these are necessary for a healthy working bowel.
3. Whole grains are a very important part of our diet. They need to be in their natural state with their fiber and nutrients intact. Look under the heading of grains and their therapeutic properties in this book, and you will see there are plenty of alternatives to white wheat flour. Drastically cut down on refined flours or better still avoid them altogether, and add a variety of whole grains mentioned later in this book.
4. Linseeds are wonderful little seeds. They are indispensable for a number of reasons. They add fiber to our diets, along with 'essential fatty acids' and, due to the fact they are mucilaginous, they have a very soothing affect on our digestive tract. The opposite is true of bran. They are a very rich source of 'omega 3' and most of us are short of this unless we eat plenty of oily fish. Research has shown they contain compounds that protect us from breast cancer (men can

also get breast cancer, although admittedly much less often). They are also good for any inflammatory conditions. Most people find them very effective in relieving constipation in a very mild and soothing way, with plenty of added bonuses.

For those few of you who find these measures are still not enough to get things moving, I suggest you see a naturopath or nutritionist. To find a practitioner swiftly, use a search engine on the Internet. Preferably look for the professional governing body in your country, to ensure you find a properly qualified person.

A case study will reveal what other measures are needed. Along with dietary changes, there could be a need for acupuncture, reflexology, or some chiropractic work or massage. Maybe you need specific supplements and/or herbs.

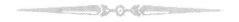

Chapter 9

Sweetness and Lite

"Jackie: Pity there's no such thing as Sugar Replacement Therapy
Victoria: There is. It's called chocolate"
Victoria Wood: Mens sana in thingummy doodah

Carbonated Drinks (Soft Or Soda Drinks)

Do you drink fizzy drinks? These drinks are usually very high in sugar with about ten spoonfuls or more in a normal can. This huge amount of sugar rushes straight into the bloodstream, which in turn causes an emergency response. The pancreas has to produce insulin to bring the blood sugar levels back down to normal. This sugar is extremely acid forming, encouraging the release of calcium from the bones to help neutralize this sudden surge in acid levels.

When you drink soft drinks containing caffeine, this effect is amplified. Soft drinks can also be highly addictive, due to their high sugar and caffeine content. It concerns me greatly when I think how much of these drinks children consume every day.

Another problem with these drinks is the fact that they are carbonated. Carbon dioxide is forced into the liquid. As we know, carbon dioxide is a waste product and contributes to higher blood acidity.

The final negative ingredient is phosphoric acid, which is also extremely acid forming. In a nutshell, soft drinks contain large amounts of sugar, often caffeine, carbon dioxide and phosphoric acid, the perfect drink for degeneration. If you have children, think about how much they are drinking. To add insult to injury they are dehydrating drinks. At this point you are probably wondering about diet drinks that are becoming ever more popular. They contain artificial sweeteners and have no place in a healthy diet, either.

Artificial Sweeteners

There are an estimated 4,000 food and drink products sweetened with artificial sweeteners.

So why would you want to consume something we call 'artificial'? Most dieters and even non-dieters use sweeteners or products containing them to avoid extra calories while still maintaining a sweet tooth. Numerous studies in both animals and humans have confirmed a very ironic fact, that artificial sweeteners increase appetite and contribute to cravings for sweet and fatty foods! One such study of 78,694 women by the American Cancer Society determined that a significantly higher percentage of artificial sweetener users gained weight than non-users! Animals fed these sweeteners become considerably fatter compared to those not fed with artificial sweeteners. Some male subjects were given artificial sweeteners or sugar, and both groups put on weight. For those taking the artificial sweeteners, it just took a little longer.

You may be surprised to hear artificial sweeteners can be very addictive, making it hard for some people to give them up. These sweeteners can become even more addictive when consumed with caffeine found in cokes, coffee, tea, and even de-caf contains some caffeine. All of this is putting considerable extra strain on the body's resources, using up reserves that would otherwise be put to better use. Anything you consume will need to be broken down by the liver into smaller components by different processes, before the body can use it or render it harmless as in the case of artificial sweeteners. When we consume nutritious foods, the body will use some of the nutrients the food provides to break down the food itself, and the rest is used for vital repair work. In the case of artificial sweeteners they provide no nutrients, but use up considerable resources to render them harmless.

Amazingly, artificial sweeteners account for a huge proportion of all non-drug complaints received by the FDA (Food and Drug Administration) in the USA. The list of complaints is long; here are just a few side effects you could experience with continual use:

~ headaches
~ tiredness
~ memory loss
~ mood swings
~ rashes

~ sleep problems

~ dizziness.

These sweeteners have been a huge success in terms of profit for the pharmaceutical companies that produce them. Used in 4,000 different products! You could be consuming more than you realize. Read the labels carefully. Americans have increased their yearly intake of low-calorie sweeteners to twenty-four pounds (11 kilos)! Still, obesity figures continue to rise. How much are you consuming? More importantly, how much are your children consuming?

Sugar

Sugar is seriously acid forming and highly addictive. It very effectively interferes with digestion. If you are going to have a sugary food occasionally then eat it on its own.

It has been estimated that the average American (Europe is never far behind most American trends) consumes about fifty teaspoons of sugar a day!!!! This is absolutely shocking.

Sugar is so addictive that most people find it hard to give it up. It's found in so many products today that, once again, you are probably consuming much more than you realize.

Consuming sugar puts an enormous strain on our immune system, as it continually evokes an auto-immune response, putting our whole system out of balance and causing it considerable extra wear and tear.

Sugar enters the bloodstream too quickly, raising our blood sugar levels. This in turn triggers the pancreas to produce insulin to bring the blood sugar levels down again. It does its job well and brings blood sugar levels down too much. This causes a yo-yo effect, making most people reach for something that will raise their blood sugar levels again - something containing sugar. Refined sugar is totally void of nutrients, and therefore our bodies will rob nutrients from other systems to enable them to deal with this constant influx.

Sugar is converted into triglycerides by the liver and then stored as fat. A lot of so-called 'low-fat' or 'no-fat' products can contain sugar instead to add flavor. These products will eventually turn to fat! Ironic don't you think?

Sugar encourages osteoporosis, as it's so highly acidic. The body will draw on its reserve of calcium to help neutralize the higher acid levels.

Food Labeling

Patients often ask me, what should I look out for on food labels? My main reply is, keep it simple. If you are eating wholesome, natural foods, there are very few labels you will need to read, and on those foods that have labels, the list will be short, with ingredients you recognize. If the label has a long list or has words you don't recognize or have difficulty pronouncing, put the product back on the shelf.

The more sugary foods we eat, the more addicted we become and the more accustomed we become to a sweet taste, and as time goes on the more we need.

Many people are totally reliant on refined sugar, plus refined flour and stimulants like tea, coffee, cokes and chocolate (that contain plenty of sugar) to give them the energy to cope throughout the day. They are in a vicious circle that is difficult to get out of. The more you rely on sugar and stimulants, the more tired you will become, the more stimulants you will use and the more deficient you will become. Eventually life becomes very hard work.

To begin the regeneration program, you will need to start cutting down on your sugar consumption. You may well be more addicted than you realize. Read labels carefully; you will be surprised where sugar crops up. Eventually, you will end up using molasses, muscovado sugar and cold-pressed honey sparingly. As time goes on, you will develop a less sweet tooth, your blood sugar levels will become stable and you will gain real energy, as you begin to get the nutrients your body needs.

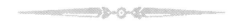

Chapter 10

Fats and Salt

"Christmas is coming, the geese are getting fat,
please put a penny in an old man's hat"
Beggar's rhyme

Fat Phobia

In our society, we mostly fall into two categories; one type eating too much fat - especially the wrong sort of fat - and then there are those who try to avoid fat at all costs, reaching for 'no-fat' or 'fat-reduced' or 'low-fat' products.

However, there are fats that are of vital importance to us. They are called 'essential fatty acids'. We must obtain these fatty acids from our food on a daily basis. They are essential for making a whole host of important hormones.

They are needed to produce all the prostanoid hormones, one of the ways cells communicate with each other. Steroid hormones are manufactured in glands like the adrenals, ovaries and testicles, whereas prostanoid hormones are produced in every cell of our bodies. All this is dependent on two 'essential fatty acids', linoleic acid and alpha-linolenic acid. We manufacture Omega-3 from alpha-linolenic acid. The majority of oils found on supermarket shelves have had alpha-linolenic acid removed, enabling the manufacturers to keep the oils on the supermarket shelves for months, even years.

Our cells need to be flexible and soft to allow substances to pass in and out, but firm enough to keep the fluid in between the cells out. At this point, we are literally what we eat. Too many saturated or damaged, processed fats in our diet produce cells that are too hard and too inflexible. This makes it more difficult for hormones, nutrients, etc to travel in and out of the cells. Essential fatty acids keep our cell membranes in good order, flexible enough to allow the correct flow in and out of the cells. What symptoms would we notice if our cells were not flexible enough? We would notice changes in our skin, hair and nails. Internal changes are harder for us to detect.

Facts on Fats

This is a huge subject, and I will try to keep it as simple as possible.

Most of the information you have received over the years has come from advertising that has been paid for by the oil and margarine industry itself. Advertising budgets can be quite substantial in an industry worth 80 billion dollars! Why wouldn't they say their products are good for us? According to Udo Erasmus, an internationally recognized authority on fats and oils (who has sifted through thousands of research papers), some fats kill and some fats heal.

Traditionally, oil pressing was a cottage industry, each large village or town having a press. Once the oil had been produced, it was handled with great care, as light, oxygen and heat would easily destroy the oil's beneficial properties. The oils were bought in small quantities, stored in dark glass bottles and kept in a cool place. They had a reasonably short shelf life unlike a lot of oils today.

Things changed and a huge industry grew. Enormous continuous-feed, screw-type, heat-producing oil presses were built to replace the small, slow, cold temperature presses. Automation made their operation highly efficient, drastically cutting labor costs. Natural nutrients are removed from the oil like carotene, Vitamin E and lecithin, making the oil 'pure'. Some synthetic antioxidants (AOs) are added to these refined oils, as the natural AOs have been removed. The shelf life has been improved for the industry's benefit, not for our health benefit.

A lot of things happen to nutritious seeds during their complicated journey to becoming colorless, tasteless oil stripped of all its nutrients.

The various stages of processing create unnatural molecules our bodies are not well equipped to handle. These fats are toxic to the body and will add to cell rigidity. These oils and fats certainly don't supply the body with the necessary raw materials to produce adequate hormones. Margarine is made from these oils by a further process, called hydrogenation. The oil is put under pressure with hydrogen gas at high temperatures, in the presence of a metal catalyst, fifty per cent nickel and fifty per cent aluminum, further damaging the oil. The oil becomes 'saturated' with hydrogen, making it solid at room temperature. These processed oils have been shown to increase cholesterol! They decrease beneficial high-density lipoprotein (HDL), interfere with our liver's detoxification system and interfere with essential fatty acid function. These oils and hydrogenated fats are used extensively in the food industry, and can be found in hundreds of manufactured food products.

The very word cholesterol instills fear. But you may or may not know that our liver produces about seventy-five per cent of our cholesterol needs, and twenty-five per cent comes from our diets. Our bodies need cholesterol for the production of estrogen, testosterone, adrenaline and Vitamin D, to name but a few. Just avoiding too many foods that contain cholesterol is only part of a much larger picture. If you avoid cholesterol foods altogether, the liver will have to produce more. Turning to margarine certainly isn't the answer. Processed vegetable oils account for seventy-four per cent of the plaque build-up in our arteries, according to the research.

'Extra Virgin' olive oil is simply cold pressed, and it does not go through numerous processes. It's an Omega-9, also know as mono-unsaturated. Research shows that this oil protects against cardiovascular disease. It has a positive effect on the brain, is associated with a lower incidence of cancer and contributes to general good health. Other cold pressed oils can be found in health shops and some supermarkets.

We eat far too many refined oils, margarine and shortenings, causing an imbalance. These refined fats that are found in thousands of products, need to be metabolized like everything else we consume. This creates an 'essential fatty acid' shortage, which are vital to our health.

There are two classes of essential fatty acids we need in our diets, Omega-3 and Omega-6. They are converted into three types of hormone-like substances. One type, called series-1 prostaglandins, has an anti-inflammatory effect, then the second type, series-2 prostaglandins, is involved in inflammation and thickening the blood. The other type is series-3 prostaglandins, which are anti-inflammatory. These three need to be in balance. These days, the balance is tipped in favor of inflammation. We eat too many processed oils and fats, too much saturated animal fat and far too little in the way of fish, wild game, raw nuts and seeds or plants rich in essential fatty acids.

If we don't eat fish or wild game, which provide EPA (eicosapentaenoic acid, which is pivotal in preventing heart disease, cancer, and many other diseases), we do have a mechanism in place that will convert alpha-linolenic acid into EPA. To enable the body to convert alpha-linolenic acid to EPA, it needs certain nutrients like Vitamin B6, Vitamin C, magnesium and zinc. Most people on an average diet don't get enough of these nutrients. The conversion can also be blocked by an excess consumption of processed oils, margarine and shortenings. Fruit, vegetables and whole grains are rich in Vitamins C and B6, magnesium and zinc.

Inflammatory conditions are common these days, and is it any wonder? Our diets are blocking our natural pathways for the production of the correct amounts of series-1 and series-3 prostaglandins that help to balance inflammatory processes and pain.

What Should We Be Eating?

To ensure we get enough 'essential fatty acids' and avoid damaged processed fats:

Take a large jar and fill with one measure each of sesame, sunflower and pumpkin seeds with two measures of flax/linseeds. Keep in the refrigerator away from light, heat and oxygen. Grind two tablespoons in a coffee grinder fresh each day and add to your

---

Omega-3

Omega-3 essential fatty acid is found mainly in marine plant life called phytoplankton and on land in linseeds. Fish such as salmon, tuna, sardines, and mackerel are our primary sources of Omega-3. It protects against heart disease by lowering LDL cholesterol. Omega-3 helps to keep the blood thin, preventing blood clots. It acts as an anti-inflammatory, making it useful for arthritis, and also helps to protect against cancer.

Wild salmon per 100 grams contains about 6.5 per cent Omega-3 fatty acid, with about six grams of fat. Farmed salmon per 100 grams contains about 0.8 per cent Omega-3 fatty acid, with about eleven grams of fat. This is a perfect example of 'You are what you eat'. The diet of the wild salmon is very different from those fed in captivity.

However, if you don't like fish, our richest source of alpha-linolenic acid in plant form is flaxseed or linseed (linseeds and flaxseeds are the same thing).

breakfast. Add to yogurt or museli (pre-soaked) or porridge once it has been cooked.

Take ½lb (225 g) of butter and allow it to soften a little, then gradually mix in 8fl oz (23 ml) of extra virgin olive oil a few drops at a time until creamy and smooth. Kept in the fridge, it will be spreadable.

· Cut down drastically on damaged processed oils and fats, found in thousands of different products, like chocolate, cakes, biscuits, pastries, etc. Get into the habit of reading labels. Study the list of ingredients carefully; it can make fascinating reading.

If you have to fry, then use a tiny amount of olive oil or sesame oil.

Eat raw nuts on a regular basis.

Cut down on meat and eat more fish (not farmed if possible), especially the oily types.

If you are on a 'very' low-fat diet, you may not be getting enough 'essential fatty acids' (vital for your metabolism and helping to break down body fat, to name but two of many functions) or adequate amounts of 'fat soluble' vitamins.

Are you getting enough 'essential fatty acids' to maintain health and vitality? The above seven simple steps will help towards making a big difference. Every small health step you take now will make the journey through life a much more pleasant one, with less complaints and discomfort later on in life.

We need to consume flaxseeds, also known as linseeds. These seeds are especially medicinal as they contain about forty per cent alpha-linolenic acid. We gain more flexibility from this oil than from any other oil derived from seeds or nuts. In second place would be oil from walnuts, but this only has about ten per cent alpha-linolenic acid. Most people think of linseed oil as a wood preserver. That's right, linseed oil gives life to dull wood and helps to preserve it. In the same way linseed will give life to a dull body and help to preserve it. It will give flexibility to cells, enabling them to function better, allowing communication between the cells by the production of prostaglandins, those prostanoid hormones we talked about earlier.

IMPORTANT: only consume linseeds and linseed oil that is fit for human consumption.

Sugar - Another Fat!!

Sugar is broken down into smaller molecules called triglycerides. What are the implications?

1. It impairs blood flow.
2. It raises the risk of coronary artery narrowing.
3. It raises insulin levels, which in turn raise our triglyceride and cholesterol levels.

Remember to read the labels of 'low-fat' or 'no-fat' products carefully, as they often contain sugar instead.

Octacosanol is derived from wheat germ. It takes ten pounds of wheat to produce 1,000 micrograms of octacosanol. This naturally derived wheat germ oil concentrate has been clinically proven to increase oxygen utilization. Found in capsule form in health shops.

Culinary Oils

You need to know some golden rules that are very important when choosing any oil.

1. Always choose cold pressed, or extra virgin oils, which have been produced without heat or chemicals. The heat and chemicals change the molecular structure of the oils, making them less than healthful.
2. Always buy only those oils found in dark glass bottles. The dark glass protects the oil from light damage. Certain plastic bottles can leach their chemicals into the oils.
3. If possible, buy organic.

If an oil isn't cold pressed or extra virgin, in dark glass bottles and preferably organic, it's likely to be highly refined.

Oils are used for:
~ salads
~ marinades
~ pouring over vegetables
~ on bread instead of butter or margarine
~ pasta sauces

~ stir-fries

~ home-made mayonnaise

~ massage.

Heating oil has a negative effect on its healthful properties. If you need to fry or cook with oil, use a tiny amount of olive oil or sesame oil.

Never allow the oil to get so hot that it smokes; if this happens don't use it.

To protect and preserve your oils better, add garlic, rosemary or thyme to them. Put some herbs into a jar and cover completely with the oil of your choice. It's important the herb is completely covered with the oil. Shake daily. Then after two weeks strain the oil and throw the herb away. For stronger tasting oil, repeat the above steps.

All your oils need storing in a cool dark place, away from the heat of your stove, and never near a sunny window.

Almond oil is expensive, used in small amounts in desserts and cookies. It takes 1,000 almonds to process just one pint of almond oil.

Bourass oil is a mixture of sunflower, wheat and borage oil. The oil has been used for centuries to regulate female hormones. Don't heat this oil, use for salads.

Canola oil is from a genetically engineered version of rapeseed, which is wild mustard. It has a bland taste. Avoid.

Corn oil is made from the germ of the corn kernel (corn on the cob).

Cottonseed oil is made from regular cottonseeds, usually used with other oils in vegetable oil products like margarine. Avoid.

Hazelnut oil is easy to digest, really good for salads, and can also be used as a massage oil.

Linseed oil has the highest linoleic acid content of any culinary oil. Never heat this oil. It needs to be handled with care. Mix with other oils in salads.

Olive oil is rich in mono-saturated but low in essential fatty acids. This oil is fairly stable and olives, being soft, are therefore easy to press. Extra virgin olive oil is one of only a few unrefined oils found in the supermarkets. Unlike most other oils, extra virgin olive oil still retains some chlorophyll, magnesium, Vitamin E, carotene and many other substances.

Peanut oil is made by pressing steamed-cooked peanuts, and can be heated to a high temperature of 440 F!! Peanuts supply one-sixth of the world's supply of vegetable oil. Avoid.

Poppy seed oil should never be heated.

Rice bran oil is made from rice polishing.

Safflower oil is made from a kind of thistle. The flowers were used in the dye industry, to produce a natural red color. The oil is a by-product.

Sesame oil is the oldest, popular throughout the Far East. The raw seeds are pressed to produce yellow oil. These seeds are easy to press without heat and contain their own natural preservatives, which help to stabilize the oil. Good for stir-fries and can be used for massage.

Sunflower oil is made from sunflower seeds. A large percentage comes from Russia.

Vegetable oil is usually made from soya beans and is cheap. This oil accounts for eighty per cent of the world's consumption. Avoid.

Walnut oil was once only used to polish violins. A lovely oil, especially in salads. Don't heat this oil.

All culinary oils contain about 120 calories per tablespoon.

The Virgin Oils I Use

For general use and cooking- I use *cold pressed* or *extra virgin olive oil* and *sesame oil.*

For salads and over vegetables, I use a mixture of *cold-pressed walnut, flax* and *olive oil* in varying degrees.

Salt

Most of us consume too much salt. It's estimated that the average person consumes about four to eight grams a day, which is far too much. You are probably eating far more than you realize. It's found in processed meat, canned foods, most cheeses, processed meals, salty snacks, tomato-based foods, etc.

There are products on the market that are lower in sodium, as they contain potassium chloride and much less sodium chloride. We should be aiming for about 2.5g a day.

You will need to start cutting down gradually, otherwise your food will seem very tasteless. Eventually, you will begin to taste the food itself, as you re-educate your taste buds. Too much sodium has been associated with fluid retention and high blood pressure.

Here is a way of adding more taste and less salt. Maybe at first, while you are weaning yourself off salt, you could use a higher proportion of salt and gradually reduce to the amount suggested below.

Salt Reducer
    1 teaspoon celery seeds
    1 tablespoon dried thyme
    1 tablespoon dried oregano
    1 tablespoon fine sea salt

Grind the herbs together into a powder and add to the salt.

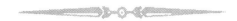

Chapter 11

Proteins

"Give me a good digestion, Lord,
and also something to digest"
Prayer, Chester Cathedral

Meat

I am often asked about meat. Some people have assumed that as a naturopath, I must be a vegetarian. However, I do eat meat and fish on occasion. I avoid beef and pork because they are the most acid forming of meats. I will eat lamb, chicken and duck. Lamb is reared in large open spaces and is grass fed. Chicken or duck, I eat preferably free-range or organic. I avoid farmed fish. If you are able to find goat's meat, that would also be fine. Goats are reared in the open, in the fresh air and eat a varied diet.

In general, vegetarians tend to be healthier than meat eaters, but not exclusively. This is due in part to the fact that many vegetarians are better informed on health matters. They eat far more vegetables, whole grains, beans, lentils, nuts and seeds, whereas most meat eaters rarely eat these types of food. Meat does have negative aspects, but so do dairy products. Some vegetarians opt for large amounts of cow's cheese and milk instead, ending up eating far too much of them. This is not a healthy alternative.

Most of the meat we find today isn't like it was years ago. Nearly half the antibiotics used in America are used on factory farm animals like pigs, cattle, chickens, turkey and fish, like farmed salmon and trout. The picture isn't a lot better in Europe, either. How much do you consume?

Intensively reared, factory-farmed animals are kept in appalling conditions - it's quite shocking. They are penned up for twenty-four hours a day, never experiencing daylight or fresh air. Often, as in the case of pigs, they live on concrete with just enough room to sit down or stand up. Where chickens are concerned, they exist in a cage with a floor space no bigger than a piece of A4 paper. These cages are stacked in a multi-storey arrangement. Factory-farmed animals are fed food laced with antibiotics, chemicals, hormones, sawdust, paper pulp, and sometimes the remains of diseased animals. Chicks are so stuffed with chemicals that they grow very fast; so fast that their immature legs don't develop fast enough to hold this huge weight gain. What are all these additives doing to us or, for that matter, to our children?

We know that while we are under stress, we produce chemicals within the body that are toxic, causing all sorts of signs and symptoms. Animals reared under these conditions show signs of great stress. What is this doing to their systems and the quality of their meat, which we in turn eat?

Reasons for Cutting Down on Meat Consumption
1. Meat is harder to digest and assimilate, compared to vegetable proteins.
2. Meat encourages an alkaline environment in the colon, which can promote the wrong bacteria, the 'unfriendly bacteria'.
3. Meat will contain added toxins, like antibiotics, hormones and pesticides (free-range or organic are better options).
4. Eating meat will put the brakes on our detoxifying processes.
5. Avoid beef and pork completely, as they are the most acid forming, and extremely difficult to digest.
6. Avoid farmed fish, which often contains high levels of chemicals.
7. Meat lacks fiber.
8. A diet high in meat can put an extra strain on the kidneys.

If you do decide to eat meat:
1. Try to buy genuine free-range, and/or organic. Unfortunately, wild game isn't so easy to find these days.
2. Eat meat in moderation.
3. Eat meat with plenty of vegetables.
4. Avoid smoked meats and most 'deli' meats.
5. Avoid anything you can't recognize. For example sausages - who knows what goes into them? Even meat pies?

However, if you are contemplating a detoxification program you will need to give up meat for just a little while.

Fish

Include deep-sea fish, fresh or frozen, in your diet. Some fish is frozen at sea as soon as it's caught.

Fish is important to our diet. It's a high-quality protein. The flesh is tender, flaky and easy to digest (if it's not overcooked). It contains 'essential fatty acids', lowering cholesterol and protecting against heart disease.

Fresh fish, once dead, rapidly becomes prone to fungal and bacterial infections, which usually cause corrosion of the skin of the fish.

A fresh fish will have:
- ~ shiny, clear, bright eyes
- ~ moist, purple gills
- ~ neat and clean body flaps
- ~ scales that are firmly attached (unless they have been removed)
- ~ an agreeable aroma, with a hint of the sea.

A stale or badly stored fish will have:
- ~ skin that appears dull and slimy to the touch
- ~ eyes that have become dull and sunken
- ~ gills that have turned gray
- ~ loose scales
- ~ a very fishy smell.

Press the fish lightly with your thumb - the flesh should bounce back if it's fresh.

Once you have purchased your fresh fish, it's best to use it almost immediately. If you want to store it for another time, you would be better off buying frozen. Once you get your fish home wash it well and cook it enough to kill any pathogens but not too much as to make it dry.

Vegetable Proteins

If you are contemplating becoming a vegetarian, or cutting down drastically on meat, remember one simple rule: when eating vegetable proteins instead of meat, you should mix beans or lentils with grains. For example, hummus (chickpea dip) with rice cakes, or lentil dip with oatcakes, or bean stew with boiled brown rice.

Beans and lentils are short of certain 'essential amino acids', and most grains are short of other essential amino acids, so mixing bean and lentils with grains will enable you to get all the essential amino acids you would get from meat and fish.

Amino Acids - What are They?
Protein must first be broken down into amino acids before the body can use them for building and repair work. Some are essential, meaning we cannot manufacture them for ourselves, whereas other amino acids can be manufactured by us. So if we remember this simple rule, we will get our full complement of essential amino acids.

~ Other sources of non-animal protein - nuts, seeds, tofu.
~ Other sources of animal protein - eggs (buy free-range or organic), yogurts, sheep and goat cheeses.

The sad fact is, the giant food companies with their enormous advertising budgets have persuaded us that their highly refined, totally processed, multi-sprayed, genetically engineered foods are actually good for us. We have one lot of multi-national companies producing food that totally undermines our health, while another set of multi-national companies waits on the sidelines to come to our rescue with a 'quick-fix' drug of one description or another.

Do you want to live with the side effects of these foods and drugs? I don't want to leave you with the impression that I am totally against the pharmaceutical industry - I'm not. However, drugs should be used as a last resort, not as a first resort.

For instance, if you have high cholesterol, you should first change your diet, and if that doesn't lower your levels, only then should you consider taking cholesterol-lowering drugs.

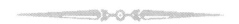

Part Two

Good Eating

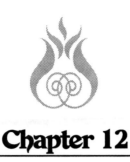

Chapter 12

Fruit and Vegetables

"An apple a day keeps the doctor away"
20th century proverb

Fresh fruit and vegetables are the most important tools of the trade. They are vital in our quest to turn our degeneration into regeneration. They are available everywhere, they are so easy to come by. Buying plenty of fresh produce need not be expensive. For those on a tight budget, there are always homegrown seasonal fruit and vegetables that are far less expensive than the more exotic imported produce that is out of season. When I say home grown I don't necessarily mean you grow them yourself, I mean grown in your area by small producers or enthusiastic gardeners who grow too much for their own needs.

Of course, organically grown produce is always better for our health and the environment but if this isn't available or beyond your budget, then wash your fruit and vegetables well and some can be peeled. At the very least avoid genetically modified and irradiated fruit and vegetables. Some people say that we should only eat organic vegetables and fruit. In a perfect world this would be ideal, however we don't live in a prefect world and plenty of well-washed non-organic fruit and vegetables are better than eating processed foods or not eating as much as you would have done because they are not organic.

People often ask me about frozen vegetables. These are not ideal, but if you are in a hurry or have run out of fresh vegetables, they are always better than no vegetables, or resorting to a refined, processed meal instead. I confess to having frozen fruit and vegetables in my freezer for occasional use.

Fruits are very cleansing and purging, whereas vegetables are restorative; the perfect partners. They are both alkalizing and require little energy to digest. It's impossible to embark on a regeneration program without them. I often hear people say they just don't like vegetables. We will explore some of the ways that will help you to get accustomed to them. Many of us have been put off in the past by 'boiled-to-death', tasteless, soggy vegetables.

Hydroponics

Hydroponics farmers grow various fruits and vegetables free of herbicides and pesticides. The plants are grown in a controlled greenhouse environment, in which the light, air, water, plant nutrients and the spacing between plants are carefully monitored in order to achieve optimal growth in the least time and at the lowest cost. The seeds are nursed from germination through maturity in an inert growing medium, through which is pumped water that contains a balanced mix of nutrients.

As the plants grow, they travel in cradle troughs along a moving conveyor belt. The cradles expand, allowing them more growing space. The overhead lamps emit three wavelengths of light, and unlike conditions outside which constantly change, the light and temperature in these greenhouses are kept constant.

If you want to make vegetables more interesting, try the following:
· Juices
· Stir-fries
· Lightly steamed
· Soups
· Salads
· Stews
· Chopped into sticks as a snack with dips

Buying
1. From the moment that fruit or vegetables are picked, they begin to lose some of their nutrients.
2. Try to buy sun-ripened, fresh-looking undamaged produce. Bruising or rough handling can destroy nutrients.

3. Many supermarkets offer pre-washed, pre-cut vegetables, salads and fruit. The cut, exposed surfaces lose nutrients very rapidly and you pay a premium. Avoid buying your produce that way, except very occasionally for convenience.

Storage

Store your fresh fruit and vegetables in the fridge (except bananas or potatoes), or in a cool place away from sunlight.

Preparation

Fruit and vegetables should be washed just before eating. Never immerse or soak your fruit and vegetables. In most cases you should not peel. The peel is a good source of fiber and nutrients. However, apples and cucumber can be sprayed and coated with a heavy wax (you can feel it and see it if you look closely), containing chemicals and would be better peeled. You will find peeling and chopping vegetables quicker and easier if you have a good quality sharp knife, well worth the investment. It will save you time in the long run.

Salads

You need to make your salads more interesting than just lettuce (not very nutritious), tomatoes and cucumber.

Use Chinese cabbage, chicory, rocket leaves, apples, pears, red lettuce, carrots, courgettes, beans, brown rice, fresh herbs, celery, spring onions, walnuts, avocado, red and yellow peppers, radishes, young fresh spinach, chives, sprouts, asparagus, artichokes, raw cauliflower, cabbage, fresh fennel, etc.

Combining the following ingredients can make a tasty and healthy salad dressing:
- Fresh lemon juice or cider vinegar
- Extra virgin oil or any combination of cold-pressed oil
- Different herbs and/or spices like ginger
- Pepper

Soups, Stews and Casseroles

You can make endless combinations with vegetables, beans or lentils or millet or quinoa or meat. There are some really tasty recipes for soups in Part Four.

Stews and casseroles can be delicious. Even if you make meat ones you can still add plenty of vegetables.

Cooking Vegetables

Boiling vegetables in water and then throwing the water away means you will be throwing the water-soluble vitamins away, such as Vitamins C and B plus selenium and potassium. Lightly steaming vegetables is healthier. There are a variety of steamers on the market. You could buy a multi-layered pot to put on the cooker top, a metal or bamboo steamer that fits over a saucepan, or an electrical steamer. Most vegetables will take between three and five minutes. Brussels sprouts may take up to ten minutes. Avoid any aluminum cookware.

Microwaving changes the molecular structure of our food, and we don't know what long-term effect this will have on our health. I know some of you will continue to use your microwaves, so at least cut down how often you use it, and avoid microwaving your food in plastic containers - use glassware instead.

Never deep-fry vegetables, as you will lose fat-soluble nutrients, such as Vitamins E and A. Stir-frying in a wok with a very small amount of sesame oil is a good way to cook vegetables quickly. For this, the vegetables need to be cut finely.

Stir-Frying

Stir-frying is a really quick, tasty and healthy way of eating vegetables.

With a little practice and the right equipment, stir-frying can be used to create a wide variety of nourishing, delicious meals. This technique evolved as a way to conserve fuel by cooking thinly sliced food quickly over high heat. The steel woks with high sides and rounded bottoms are not very efficient when used on modern cooker tops, as they are slow and give uneven cooking results. The best type of wok is a cast iron one, which distributes and holds the heat evenly throughout the cooking process.

Ingredients must be added to the pan in order of relative cooking time, with longer cooking items added first. All the ingredients must be prepared just before you start cooking. For this the vegetables need to be cut finely, and the meat sliced thinly. Uncooked seafood, fish, poultry or meat are stir-fried first, removed while all the other ingredients are cooked, then added back at the end.

Use a teaspoon to a tablespoon of cold-pressed sesame oil or extra virgin olive oil. Don't over cook the vegetables; they should be just *al-dente*, a little crunchy.

The following is a list of suggested ingredients:
· almost any vegetable
· some fruits like pineapple
· spices and herbs like ginger, lemon grass, coriander
· sprouts
· chicken
· fish
· tofu

Individual Fruits and Vegetables

Firstly, all fruits and vegetables are bursting with vitamins, minerals, enzymes, phyto-chemicals and fiber.

Below I have listed only a few individual fruits and vegetables, to give you a brief idea about how therapeutic they can be. I have not listed all the vitamins, minerals, phyto-chemicals and enzymes in each fruit and vegetable. I advise you to eat as big a variety each week as you possibly can. Each plant has its own therapeutic properties, as you will discover below. We need them all in varying degrees.

Vegetables

Beetroot is good for nourishing the blood and increasing its oxygen capacity. A good intestinal cleanser, it also detoxifies the liver and the gallbladder. Buy fresh beetroot for use in juices and salads. Do not buy beetroot in vinegar.

Broccoli is a rich source of iron and calcium, beta-carotene, magnesium, plus many more. It has anti-cancer properties, cleanses the intestines, stimulates the liver, and contains powerful antioxidants.

Cabbage contains Vitamin U, named after it was discovered to contain ulcer-healing properties. Also contains Vitamins C and A. There are many types of cabbage - red, white or green with smooth or crinkled leaf, not forgetting Chinese cabbage. Some people find eating cabbage raw or cooked causes too much wind. Then juiced cabbage may well solve this problem. Cabbage is a rich source of minerals like calcium, potassium and sulfur. There has been some success with treating people with stomach ulcers by consuming cabbage juice for its Vitamin U content. Red cabbage contains more calcium and Chinese cabbage causes less wind than the other varieties. Cabbage helps to speed up a sluggish GI tract.

Carrots are well known for helping the liver, aiding the removal of any stagnant bile. Carrots are high in carotenes, a really good source of Vitamin A and powerful antioxidants. Carrots are good in juices, cut into sticks as snacks, grated raw in salads, steamed or put into stews and soups. Give raw carrots to children to chew on.

Celery has strong cleaning and alkalizing properties; a good blood cleanser. It can aid digestion and is a good source of magnesium. Celery helps our nervous systems and cleanses uric acid from our muscles and joints, which is helpful in arthritic conditions. It's also a good diuretic, helping to remove excess fluid from our bodies. If you have any aches and pains or fluid retention this vegetable is a good one to add to your routine. The stalks of celery should be fresh enough that they snap easily. Look up the seeds under Herbs and Spices in Part Four - they also have therapeutic properties.

Chlorophyll is the substance that makes plants green - found in green supplements like algae, chlorella, and spirulina. Also found in spinach, broccoli, rocket, dark green cabbage, etc. It is a rich source of magnesium and other minerals, has cleansing and alkalizing properties, and can help with anemia.

Cucumber is a cooling plant, an excellent diuretic and mild laxative. It dissolves uric acid, helps digestion and regulates blood pressure. It is very alkaline forming, a non-starchy vegetable, or more correctly, herb.

Chop up cucumber and fresh mint very small and add to some natural yogurt. This makes the perfect complement for hot curries, as it's very cooling.

Ginger, Onions and Garlic, combined in stir-fries, soups, salads etc, have a have powerful healing and cleansing effect on our systems. Look up the individual properties of ginger and garlic under the 'herbs and spices' section.

Onions; there are two types - strong and mild - and both come in four different colors, red, yellow, white and brown. The white onions are the mildest. Onions are one of the earliest-known food medicines, used for hundreds of years for colds. For coughs - chop up an onion finely and allow it to stand in some honey overnight. In the morning, strain and use as a cough medicine. Onions contain large amounts of sulfur, which is good for the liver.

Root vegetables, like celeriac, parsnips, sweet potatoes, yams, carrots and turnips, have good cleansing properties. They are full of nutrients and help to support many of our organs and systems.

Watercress is a diuretic, and helps to break up kidney and bladder stones. This plant is high in iodine, supporting the thyroid. It's very important to wash this plant really well.

Fruit

Apples contain pectin, which has the ability to absorb plenty of fluids from the intestines, acting like a very mild, non-irritating laxative. They help to stimulate our peristaltic movement, aiding natural bowel elimination. Apples are good for cleansing the blood, and the lymph. They are also rich in Vitamin C, B, and A.

Apricots contain powerful antioxidants, high in calcium, magnesium, beta-carotene, potassium, Vitamin C. The cobalt they contain helps in the treatment of anemia. Dried apricots contain six times more fruit sugar than the fresh variety. Dried apricots that have been soaked in water, cooked and then pureed can make a good substitute for sugar in cooking and baking.

Bananas are really good snacks, you can take them anywhere, are easy to eat and come in their own easy-to-remove packaging that is biodegradable. They are a good source of starch. They have anti-fungal, antibiotic properties. They have a mild laxative effect, help to heal ulcers, lower cholesterol and remove toxins from the body. They are high in potassium and tryptophan (good for calming the brain). If you suffer from insomnia, take a natural yogurt with a mashed banana in the evening, and avoid stimulants. Bananas are also rich in Vitamin C, K, and B6.

Blueberries are really good for the eyes, improve circulation, cleanse the blood, contain antioxidants and act as a mild laxative.

Cherries have antispasmodic properties and a natural antiseptic. They are a really good source of iron, a wonderful blood tonic. They help the body rid itself of toxic waste. They support the gall bladder and liver.

Cranberries. The Pilgrims called them crane berries, maybe because the flowers crane their necks or because cranes are very fond of them? Long before researchers found a special compound in cranberries that seemed to act as a urinary antiseptic, by preventing bacteria from coating the surface of the cells in the bladder and urinary tract, American Indian women had used cranberries for this very purpose.

Grapefruit served at the beginning of a meal will help in the digestion of meat, increase digestive enzymes and aid in the absorption of nutrients. Fresh grapefruit juice is a powerful cleanser, but be careful not to consume too much at first. It helps to remove excess mucus build-up.

Kiwifruit contains digestive enzymes and helps the body to remove excess sodium. It has more Vitamin C than oranges.

Lemons (see also under herbs and spices). They are one of the most alkalizing foods there is, making them a very useful tool for regeneration and cleansing. A simple way to take lemon therapeutically is to squeeze half a lemon, add the juice to a little warm water and drink first thing in the morning before you eat or drink anything. This will encourage the liver to cleanse and help to create a more alkaline environment. Choose lemons that are a rich, deep yellow color, that are firm but not hard. Avoid shriveled ones, or ones that have been damaged.

Lemon juice can be used instead of vinegar in salad dressings. Add a squeeze of lemon to your drinking water to add interest. A little can be added to your fruit/vegetable juices if you want.

Lemons are also a rich source of Vitamin C and potassium. I always add some fresh lemon juice to my fruit salads instead of vinegar.

Melons are full of fluid, making them good for rehydration. They are ideal for cleansing. In the summer they are perfect for quenching your thirst, especially watermelon.

Papaya contains papain, an excellent digestive aid. It has powerful anti-cancer properties, soothes intestinal inflammation and detoxifies in general. It's a good source of calcium, magnesium, Vitamin C and beta-carotene.

Pears contain iodine, which is good for the correct functioning of the thyroid. This fruit has diuretic properties, making it good for fluid retention.

Pineapple contains bromelain, a really good digestive enzyme. Taken regularly, they can help to prevent bacteria and parasites.

Raspberries help to remove excess mucus from our systems. They are good for the health of the female reproductive system, especially for menstrual cramps.

Strawberries have antiviral, anti-cancer and antibacterial properties.

Organic produce is food grown without the use of insecticides, herbicides, artificial fertilizers and growth-stimulating chemicals/hormones.

After looking through this list, I hope I have convinced you to eat a lot more fresh fruit and vegetables. They are vital to our health and help to prevent or delay the onset of chronic diseases that plague our modern society.

Fruit Bowl

Keep a well-stocked fruit bowl and place it in a prominent place. There are times when you will want to snack and taking fruit is always a better option to biscuits or chocolate or crisps. Besides, an interesting fruit selection might encourage other members of the family to eat more fresh fruit. If some of the fruit becomes a little soft don't throw it away - use it for making a juice.

Juicing

I am a great fan of juicing. It's such a good therapeutic tool. The only drawback is that the juicing machine takes a bit of cleaning. Personally I still find it less hassle than emptying the dishwasher.

Juicing is a powerful cleansing and healing tool. These juices are bursting with easy to digest and, most importantly, easy to absorb nutrients. They are extremely therapeutic, enabling you to consume concentrated enzymes. For this reason, be gentle with your system and gradually increase your consumption.

To make enzyme, co-enzyme and phyto-chemical rich drinks, you will need to invest in a 'juice extractor'. These machines are easy to find in most electrical stores. Buy the best one you can afford; they vary in price, and generally, the more expensive, the more juice they will extract from the fruit and vegetables. The fruit and vegetables are always used raw, never cooked.

The fruit and vegetables are not usually peeled, only washed and chopped. Exceptions would be the skin of pumpkins, squashes and melons, especially watermelons, as their skins are too tough to go through the machine. Pips found in, for example, apples and pears don't need removing, only large stones like those found in peaches are removed beforehand. I would not juice a banana, as it's far too starchy. Use them in a blender, but more on that later.

Juicing isn't a replacement for eating plenty of fresh fruit and vegetables (except for those of you that hate eating fruit and vegetables). Juicing is meant to be as well as, a way of getting extra support for cleansing and healing. For this reason it's important to throw the pulp away, or make it into compost for the garden. If you consume the pulp you are defeating the whole object of juicing in the first place.

Fruit and vegetables can be juiced together. A good combination would be about seventy per cent vegetables and thirty per cent fruit, up to a fifty-fifty mix. An all-fruit juice isn't a good idea, as it enters the bloodstream too quickly, raising our blood sugar levels. If you have children that like fruit juices, then dilute with fifty per cent water for them and for yourself. This is a case where fruit juice with the same quantity of fizzy water would be better than giving your children squashes or fizzy drinks. However, if you prefer, you could juice with vegetables only.

The juice should be made fresh every time. As soon as the juice has been made, it starts to deteriorate quite quickly, as oxygen and light start to break down nutrients and especially enzymes. The general rule is to drink the juice there and then for maximum benefit. Everything in life has degrees, so drinking a fresh juice a couple of hours later is still better than not drinking any. If, for instance, you decide to send your children to school with a juice, then put it in a thermos flask to minimize the damage.

Juices are used to boost our body's cleansing and healing processes, so go easy at first. These juices are concentrated with vitamins, minerals and enzymes in a form the body can easily utilize with little effort, so you don't want to encourage cleansing faster than the body can handle. One large glass at least four times a week would be a very good way of topping up our enzyme levels, along with a good diet. As a more effective tool for cleansing, you should work your way up to drinking a full glass one to three times a day.

During the course of a week, you should try to get as big a variety of fruit and vegetables as possible. If you can't get organic produce, then make sure you wash non-organic produce thoroughly. You can buy special liquids designed for washing fruit and vegetables properly. If you hate eating vegetables, it's definitely worth juicing them, as most people end up really liking juices. You might surprise yourself. Try adding mint or cinnamon or ginger or lemon juice to enhance the taste. I am sure you will find combinations you will like.

N.B. If you have a serious condition, I advise you to see your doctor or naturopath before deciding to embark on a serious juicing program for detoxifying and regenerating.

Blending

This could be a way of getting children to take fresh fruit and proteins like yogurt or tofu. It's especially good for children who don't like eating breakfast. This will help to nourish them and keep their blood sugar more stable, compared to the usual sugary breakfasts or to eating nothing at all.

Kids' Power Packs

Banana Smoothie
  Yogurt or tofu
  Bananas
  Carob
  Honey
  Place all ingredients together in a blender.
  If necessary add soya milk, rice milk or oat milk.
  Blend well.

Fruity Smoothie
  Yogurt or tofu
  fresh fruit, like berries
  honey to taste
  Place all ingredients in a blender.
  Add soya, oat, or rice milk if the mixture is too thick.

Carob Smoothie
  Yogurt or tofu
  Carob powder

Honey to taste

Place all ingredients together in a blender.

Add soya, oat, or rice milk if the mixture is too thick.

Soup for Children

Children will often eat soups if they cannot detect any vegetable bits. This is where a blender works wonders. Use some of the more colorful, sweeter vegetables like pumpkins, carrots or parsnips with coconut milk.

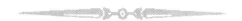

Chapter 13

Yogurts, Grains and Seeds

"Food is an important part of a balanced diet"
Fran Lebowitz: Metropolitan Life

Yogurt

The beneficial bacteria in yogurts keep the body's digestive system working correctly. Use only natural 'live' yogurt. If you need to take a course of antibiotic treatment, make sure you eat plenty of yogurt every day for a few weeks after treatment, and take some pro-biotic capsules or powder, available from health shops. Antibiotics indiscriminately destroy both our 'unfriendly bacteria' and our 'friendly bacteria'. Yogurts will help to reintroduce some of the beneficial bacteria.

Eating yogurts on a regular basis will help to keep certain yeasts such as candida from multiplying to harmful levels. If you are dairy intolerant, you will find you can eat natural 'live' yogurts as long as they contain active cultures, as they break down and pre-digest the lactose for us.

Take care to make sure your yogurt is purely a 'live' yogurt with nothing added. A little while ago, I was in the supermarket, reaching for my usual yogurts, when a representative asked me to try a famous yogurt drink instead. However, on the label of this natural yogurt drink was - yogurt, skimmed milk (which doesn't contain the bacteria we are looking for), sugar and dextrose (a form of sugar)! Remember, sugar turns to fat and encourages our 'unfriendly bacteria'.

I can hear some of you saying how you hate natural yogurts. Most people I have asked to eat them end up loving them.

- Chop up a load of fruit, place in a bowl and add the yogurt with seeds and nuts.
- Add yogurt to your muslin, which has dried fruit, nuts and seeds in it. Muslin must be soaked overnight in water before you eat it. This ensures the activation of enzymes, making it much easier for us to digest. It also allows the muslin to swell in the bowl and not in our stomachs. This is important.

> When volunteers ate six ounces of yogurt daily for a year, those who ate 'live' cultures had twenty-five per cent fewer colds and ten times fewer symptoms of hay fever and allergies, than those who ate yogurt with 'dead' cultures.
>
> Fermented milk products have been used for centuries. Today, it's easy to find many varieties of natural 'live' yogurts that can be organic or even made from sheep and goat's milk.

Home-Made Yogurts

It's easy to find electric yogurt makers. Making yogurts this way is simple and cheap. I also find they taste better.

Follow the manufacturer's instructions. The machines are thermostatically controlled, making it easy to use. With this method, you can use a large tablespoonful from your previously homemade yogurt. This can be done about ten times before you need to buy another shop bought one.

Two Basic Methods

The first method uses fresh milk - cow's milk is fine, but better still is goat or sheep's milk. Take one liter of fresh milk, bring almost to the boil and keep on heat for fifteen minutes. Cool the milk rapidly to 43 to 45°C or 110 to 112°F by placing the pan in a sink of cold water. Mix a large heaped tablespoon of yogurt with a little of this milk, then add to the bulk of the milk and mix well.

The second method uses dried milk from cows, but goat or sheep would be better. Use boiled water to mix with the powder (to manufacturer's instructions) and leave to cool. Mix a heaped tablespoon of yogurt with a little milk, then add to the bulk of the milk and mix well. If you would like your yogurt a little creamier, add a bit more dried milk.

This is the only time you should use cow's milk (though the other milks are better), as the making process pre-digests milk.

One heaped tablespoon of making to one liter of milk is usually sufficient. Too much will overcrowd the making and it will be lumpy, too little and too thin.

Leave the mixture in a warm environment, undisturbed. The process can take up to eight hours, depending on the method used. If you are making it for the first time, check from time to time to see how long the making is taking to set. Do this carefully without disturbing it too much.

This method works well, but I would advise you to buy a making-making machine if you are going to be making large quantities.

Grains

Grains are grasses which all produce edible seeds, or kernels, with four basic features in common. The outer husk or hull is generally not edible and is removed. Bran, which is rich in fiber, is the inner husk; the endosperm is the starchy center, rich in carbohydrates, and the germ contains enzymes, minerals, vitamins and fatty acids.

What are whole grains? They are grains that are as nature intended - they have the endosperm, fiber and germ left intact, retaining the nutrients. Refining grains removes the fiber and the germ plus considerable amounts of enzymes, vitamins and minerals.

Gluten is a sticky protein found in wheat, rye, barley and oats. It's a very difficult substance to digest. Wheat contains much more than the other grains, with rye next and oats containing the least. Gluten has unique elastic properties, much like chewing gum, which makes pastry- and bread-making easy. This gluten can stretch to provide a honeycomb of cells capable of containing the gas from yeast as bread rises. Until recent times, barley bread was universal in the colder parts of Britain. From the eighteenth century, oats become more popular, and wheat from the nineteenth century. Wheat is now overused, we all eat too much of it, often morning, noon and night, seven days a week. For a lot of people, wheat is the only grain they eat, yet there are so many other grains that need to be included in our diets. Whole grains, of course.

Phytic acid is found in high levels in wheat and soya beans. It can chelate (combine) with at least five highly significant minerals needed for a number of enzymes systems, and make them biologically unavailable. For example, phytic acid can combine with iron, zinc, calcium, magnesium and manganese, plus others. There are other inhibitors in various foods setting up a chain reaction, depressing enzymes, causing the pancreas more work to redress the levels, but none are eaten as often as wheat.

A lot of people are told they are wheat-intolerant, and is it any wonder, when you stop to consider how much is being consumed, and its very nature.

1. It's most often eaten with most of the nutrients and fiber removed (white flour).
2. It's heavily sprayed, unless you buy organic.
3. It contains a lot of gluten that is very difficult to digest. A hundred or so years ago wheat did not contain as much gluten, but over the years it has been developed to contain more.
4. We consume far too much of it, several times a day, seven days a week, setting up problems.
5. It's very acid-forming.

Amaranth (gluten-free) is similar to quinoa, a small round seed, pale in color. It was used by the ancient Aztecs as a valuable food. Recently, it has been discovered that in areas of Africa and Latin America where it's consumed, malnutrition is rare. This is because of its high nutritional value and its ability to thrive in very poor soil, even in drought situations. This poses the question, why isn't it grown more? Amaranth is a slightly more expensive seed/grain; however, it's a concentrated food, high in protein and calcium. It's high in lysine, an amino acid that is low in wheat and most other grains. It contains more calcium and the necessary supporting nutrients like magnesium and silicon than milk. It's a rich source of fiber, easy and quick to cook, a good rice substitute, and can be used in breads, cakes, soups and grain dishes. It pops like popcorn or can be sprouted for salads. It has a mild, nutty flavor. Some health shops sell puffed amaranth as a breakfast cereal, with nothing added.

Barley (contains some gluten). Looks a little like brown rice. Whole barley contains more nutrients than the commonly used 'pearl' variety, including more fiber, twice the calcium and three times the iron. The whole grain can be boiled in water, then strained and drunk as a tea. The tea will relieve summer heat, tiredness and aid the digestion. It's soothing to the digestive tract and liver, heals stomach ulcers and lowers cholesterol. Barley can be used in soups and casseroles, or used instead of rice, or ground as flour in bread.

Buckwheat (gluten-free) has nothing to do with wheat. Buckwheat is actually a seed. The whole grain has an odd shape, triangular with a slight brown/pink color. It's a good source of rutin, which strengthens the capillaries and blood vessels, reduces blood pressure and increases circulation to the hands and feet. It contains lysine, an essential amino acid not always present in grains. There is evidence that buckwheat may help keep glucose levels under control better than other carbohydrates. Traditionally, buckwheat flour is used for making crepes (pancakes). The whole grains can be boiled and used in salads or soups.

Bulgur wheat (contains gluten) is wheat that has been partly cooked, dried and cracked. Bulgur wheat is often used in Middle Eastern cooking, in dishes like tabouleh and pilaf. Remember it's a wheat product and should be avoided if you have any problems with wheat, or are on a therapeutic diet or if you are trying to cut down. Use amaranth, quinoa, or millet instead.

Couscous (contains gluten) made from granular semolina wheat. Avoid if you are wheat intolerant or are on a therapeutic diet, or if you want to cut down on the amount of wheat you eat. Use amaranth, millet or quinoa instead, they all make very good substitutes.

Corn (gluten-free) also known as maize (corn on the cob). Native Americans traditionally cooked corn with lime. When other cultures first began using corn as a staple in the nineteenth and twentieth centuries, it resulted in an often-fatal disease called pellagra, which caused wasting away. This was due to corn not having much niacin (B3). The old secret of adding lime increased the absorption of niacin. This will not become a problem to us if we eat a varied diet. Corn is a good tonic for the kidneys and the urinary system in general. This is especially true of the corn silk that can be infused and used as a tea.

Buy the whole grain to make popcorn. Popcorn makers are cheap to buy and very easy to use, and children love them. Alternatively, use a large pan, preferably with a glass lid so that you (and the kids) can watch the process.

Corn meal is yellow, ground from the whole grain. Avoid cornstarch, which is white and refined. Corn meal is used for making polenta, recipes for which can be found in most Italian cookbooks.

Kamut (contains some gluten) is an ancient form of durum-related wheat. It flourished in Egypt more than 5,000 years ago. Grown until the Second World War, when it became almost extinct in favor of the hybrid we know as wheat today. Fortunately, seeds were recovered from some ancient burial crypts, and now organic kamut grows in Montana. This is another grain that is well tolerated by those who have problems with conventional wheat, or those who want to avoid eating so much. It makes a good substitute for wheat for bread making.

Millet (gluten-free), a very small round seed that is pale in color, looks similar to quinoa and amaranth. It's known as 'the queen of grains'. Millet is alkaline-forming and anti-fungal; one of the best grains for those with candida. It's gluten free and easily digested. It's a low-allergenic food and a good source of magnesium, potassium and Vitamin B3. Millet can be used instead of couscous, instead of breadcrumbs for stuffing, instead of rice, and the flakes can be used in muesli.

Oats (contain some gluten, but much less than wheat) are one of the richest sources of silicon, which help to renew the bones and all connective tissue. It removes cholesterol from the digestive tract and the arteries, and strengthens the cardiac muscles. It's a good source of calcium, magnesium, iron, phosphorus, manganese, Vitamin B5 and folic acid. The high fiber content has a mild laxative effect, making it excellent for indigestion, wind and an upset stomach. It's most conveniently taken in the form of porridge or muesli (remember to pre-soaked in a little water overnight). They are used to make oat cakes, easily found in supermarkets. Some are completely wheat-free and salt-free.

Quinoa (gluten-free) is a cousin of amaranth, and has some of the same amazing qualities. It was one of the staples of the Incas and was called 'the mother grain' and, though not a true grain, it is used as one. It has grown in the South American Andes for thousands of years, and thrives in high cold altitudes. Quinoa has more calcium than milk. It's a good source of iron, phosphorus, B Vitamins and Vitamin E. It looks like millet, and it's hard to tell them apart, except quinoa is slightly darker. It has a mild taste and cooks like rice in about eight to ten minutes.

Rice (gluten-free) is a staple for more than half the world's population.

Brown rice is a good source of magnesium, phosphorus, potassium, iron, manganese, Vitamin B3, Vitamin B6, folic acid and fiber, unlike white rice. It's a tropical grain and can alleviate the irritability associated with summer heat.

White rice has had the outer layer that lies directly beneath the hull removed during milling. The bit that is removed is rich in protein, fiber (soluble and insoluble), minerals, Vitamin B and Vitamin E, which help to strengthen the immune system. This outer layer is used to produce vitamin-rich concentrates and rice oil. You would be much better off eating the whole grain (brown rice). Several of the varieties listed below come in whole grain/brown rice variety. Brown rice flour can be used in all sorts of recipes with other flours.

Did You Know?

·   White rice has such a low fiber content that it only takes an hour to digest! It will raise your blood sugar levels.

·   Fifty per cent of the world's rice is eaten within eight miles of where it's grown.

·   Archaeologists have traced the cultivation of rice back at least 5,000 years.

Rye (contains gluten) is a very hard grain and is ideally suited to sourdough baking, which adds a slightly sour taste and a natural bitter taste, making it effective for the liver. This grain contains less gluten than wheat. Ii is a good source of iron, magnesium, phosphorus, potassium, zinc, manganese and Vitamin E. It's easy to find a hundred per cent sourdough rye bread in supermarkets. I have even seen organic.

Spelt (contains some gluten) is a relative of wheat. It originated in Southeast Asia and was brought to the Middle East more than 5,000 years ago, and has since spread over Europe. Very recently spelt has enjoyed a comeback in Europe, as it makes great bread. Most people who have problems with wheat, generally don't have them with spelt, which is usually well tolerated. Where any recipe calls for whole-wheat, use spelt instead. Spelt is more nutritious. It grows a hard thick husk that protects the grain from pollutants and insects, and for this reason it needs far less pesticides or other chemicals. This is good news for us, and our environment.

Triticale (contains gluten) is the first man-made grain, and is a hybrid of wheat and rye. It's a rich source of lysine, an essential amino acid often missing in other grains, but found in many other foods.

Doesn't it make you wonder, with so many grains to choose from that are so highly beneficial to our health, why the world is full of wheat? Wheat in the form of white flour products that are totally detrimental to our health?

Here are some different combinations of grains that can be used instead of wheat flour for making breads, cakes, pancakes, biscuits and pastries.

Long grain rice is four or five times as long as it is wide. An all-purpose grain, it stays separate, light and fluffy when cooked.

Medium grain rice is plump but not round. When cooked, this grain is more moist and tender than long grain.

Short grain rice is almost round in shape. The grains are softer than the above two and tend to stick together when cooked. This rice is good for sushi and rice pudding.

Arborio rice from Italy's Po Valley is a superior variety used for making risotto. A short, shiny, pearly-smooth grain that gradually absorbs hot broth when patiently stirred for forty-five minutes.

Basmati rice is fragrant, an aromatic rice from India and Pakistan. Its long slender grains have a distinctively nutty taste and it's the rice of choice with curries.

Spanish rice is a medium grain grown in Valencia, and is the one to select for paella.

Instant rice is pre-cooked and dried. The grains are cracked to allow the water to enter, so that they cook almost instantly. It has little taste and nutrients are lost. Avoid this rice.

Wild rice isn't actually rice; it's a marsh grass, a long, slender black grain. It's indigenous to North America and traditionally known as manomen, or 'water grass', and was a staple of the Ojibwat, Chippewa and Winnebago Indians.

GRAINS FOR USE INSTEAD OF WHEAT FLOUR	
Barley flour	Makes a sticky loaf. Use fifty per cent with other flours
Buckwheat flour	Makes good winter bread, dark and heavy. Mix with rice or spelt flour
Kamut flour	Can substitute a hundred per cent for whole wheat
Millet flour	Always combine with other flours, especially spelt and kamut (one third millet and two thirds other flours)
Oat flour	Light in texture, adds moisture. Use twenty per cent
Rice flour	Makes a sweeter, smoother bread. Use up to twenty per cent
Rye flour	Use fifty per cent with spelt, rice and kamut
Soy flour	Hard to digest; use only a small amount in combination with other flours
Spelt flour	Can substitute a hundred per cent for whole wheat

Seeds

Most people would never consider eating seeds every day, yet they contain 'essential fatty acids' vital to our overall health. They are also high in fiber. Add pumpkinseeds, linseeds, sunflower seeds and sesame seeds to your breakfast in muesli, porridge (once it is cooked), etc.

Seeds should not be roasted. The reason is that the food industry uses very high temperatures. The delicate and highly beneficial 'essential fatty acids' in nuts and seeds are altered or destroyed by these high levels of heat. This can turn a healthy 'fatty acid', essential to your well-being, into a health hazard. The section on 'Facts on Fats' explains why it's so important to buy oils produced by the cold pressed method.

To get the most health-giving properties from nuts and seeds, eat them raw. Avoid them if they have been roasted, blanched, salted, ground, sliced or crushed. The best-case scenario would be to buy nuts in their shells and crack them yourself. The shells keep the nuts and seeds fresh the way nature intended, reducing the likelihood of damage from light and oxygen. Another benefit from having to shell your nuts and seeds is that it certainly slows down those who find it hard not to eat a bucket load once they get going.

However, for convenience, buy shelled nuts and seeds with as long a shelf-life as possible and then keep them in the fridge. Some recipes will have nuts and seeds included for cooking. Home cooking generally uses lower temperatures than the food industry. For instance, add cashews to stir-fries and Indian cooking at the end of cooking just to warm them up. Baking with seeds and nuts occasionally is okay. However, for daily consumption seeds and nuts should be raw.

Alfalfa seeds are very tiny. They can help to reduce inflammation and aid detoxification. They are good sources of calcium, magnesium, potassium and manganese.

They are very easy to sprout. Avoid if you have lupus. For more information, look under the 'Herbs and Spices' section in Part Four.

Flaxseeds (*Linseeds*) are very small shiny seeds that are either yellow or brown. They are really good at alleviating constipation and bloating, helping to eliminate toxic waste from the bowels, and helping to strengthen the blood. They have anti-inflammatory and anti-cancer properties.

Flaxseeds are a very rich land plant source of Omega-3 and Omega-6 essential fatty acids. Most rich sources of Omega-3 come from oily fish. Flaxseeds are also a very good source of potassium, magnesium, calcium, iron, Vitamin B3 and Vitamin E. These seeds are very soothing to the digestive tract, due to their mucilaginous properties. They contain lignins, compounds that help to protect against breast cancer.

Flaxseeds can be eaten in the following ways:
· 	As they are, dry and intact
· 	Soaked in some water overnight (don't rinse in the morning)

· Ground a little in a coffee grinder
· Boiled in water - then drink the liquid.

Pumpkin seeds are green, flat and oval shaped. They are excellent for the health of the prostate gland. They can help remove intestinal parasites. Pumpkin-seed oil is a rich source of 'essential fatty acids'. They contain calcium, magnesium, zinc and B Vitamins.

Psyllium seeds are used as a laxative and intestinal cleanser. They relieve auto-toxemia caused by constipation and bacterial/fungal infection. They contain calcium, magnesium, phosphorus, potassium and zinc. Flaxseeds have a similar effect.

Sesame seeds are tiny, pale-colored seeds. They strengthen the heart, the cardiovascular system and the nervous system. They contain lignins, which act like antioxidants. Also, they inhibit cholesterol absorption from the diet. A rich source of calcium, iron, magnesium, zinc, Vitamin E, folic acid, potassium, copper, Omega-3 and six essential fatty acids.

Tahini is made by grinding sesame seeds, and is sold in jars, just like peanut butter. It's often used in dips like hummus (chickpea spread). You will find a recipe in Part Four.

Sprouting

Any type of lentils, grains, seeds and beans (except soy or aduki beans) can be sprouted easily. If you start on soybeans you might get put off, as they are the most difficult to sprout. In my experience, aduki beans can easily go mouldy, especially in warmer weather. As a beginner, try mung beans (little round green beans) first, as they are very easy to sprout.

During sprouting, vitamins, minerals and enzymes are dramatically increased. Everything that has lain dormant bursts into life.

Sprouting is a very easy and economical way of having fresh food on hand all year round, summer or winter, adding enzymes to our diets. The process is so easy that even a child can do it. The sprouting process pre-digests substances in the beans, lentils and grains, making them much easier for us to digest, assimilate and metabolize. This makes them an ideal food for those who have trouble digesting grains and beans normally. Sprouts are perfect for salads, can be added to soup (once the soup has been cooked) or to stir fries at the end of cooking.

How to Grow Sprouts

Soak one part beans or grains to three parts water overnight. In the morning, drain and rinse them well, then place them in large jars. Cover the mouth of the jar with a piece of cloth and secure with a rubber band. The piece of cloth should be very porous, like netting or gauze.

Rinse the beans or seeds twice a day through the cloth, and drain well each time. In very hot weather, it helps to rinse them three times a day; otherwise rinse morning and night, for two reasons: first, so the beans/grains don't dry out, and secondly, to prevent them going moldy. Set the jar aside on the kitchen surface, near to the sink to remind you.

Once sprouted, rinse and drain really well, put in the fridge and eat as soon as possible. Eat sprouts raw in salads, or slightly cooked. Too much cooking will destroy the enzymes, which will defeat the object.

The time it takes to sprout will vary a lot depending on how warm it is, and what you have chosen to sprout. For instance, alfalfa could take up to five days to sprout, and mung beans or fenugreek seeds could take less, depending on the time of year.

If you want to produce more sprouts more often, then you can buy a purpose-made sprouting gadget, usually made in plastic. They usually come in layers, enabling you to sprout different seeds or grains on each layer. Sprouts have some powerful cleansing properties, which can be dampened down a little if you lightly steam them.

If you are someone who feels the cold, I suggest you lightly steam your sprouts in the winter. The sprouting process changes the bio-availability of the nutrients, making them very easy to digest and assimilate. They contain compounds that assist the liver.

Sprouted Grain Bread

If you have an allergy to wheat, rye, barley or oats, sprouting is a perfect option. Sprouted wheat and rye very seldom produce any symptoms, so they can be used to make sprouted wheat/rye bread. The sprouts are dried in the sun, in a food dehydrator or in an oven at a very low temperature. Then they are ground in a blender or flourmill. Use this flour in the same way you would use any flour.

To make your own sprouted wheat or rye flour, take 800g of the whole-grains and sprout until they are about an inch long. Grind them in a meat grinder - both manual and electric grinders are quite inexpensive.

There is a recipe for sprouted bread in Part Four. If you prefer an easy life, sprouted grain breads can be bought from most health shops.

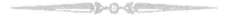

Chapter 14

Nuts and Pulses

"I had a little nut tree, nothing would it bear,
but a silver nutmeg, and a golden pear"
Nursery rhyme

Nuts

Nuts should always be eaten raw, as heat will destroy their health-promoting properties. Almonds are one of the best nuts, but other nuts are also very nutritious. They are high in B Vitamins and especially in Vitamin E. Nuts are a rich source of protein, as well as 'essential fatty acids'. The protein from nuts is easier to digest than that from meat. They are rich in linoleic acid, making them beneficial to our heart and circulatory system.

Almonds These trees grow principally in the Mediterranean, but are also cultivated in other parts of the world. If you are unable to buy them with their shells, then make sure they still have their thick brown skin. Do not buy them blanched (skins have been removed with a heat process). A rich source of calcium, magnesium, zinc, some Vitamin Bs and Vitamin E. They are also a good source of protein and are alkaline forming.

Cashews are kidney-shaped nuts, originally from India, but now cultivated in Africa and South America. These nuts are good for teeth and gums. They are high in calcium, magnesium, iron and zinc. They are only sold shelled.

Coconuts grow on palms, thriving in tropical areas. The fat from coconut is mainly saturated, but does contain magnesium and potassium. Coconut can help the thyroid along with other measures.

Pine nuts are found in the Mediterranean on certain pine trees. Pine nuts are high in protein and essential fats. They are used in many vegetarian recipes. They are a rich source of magnesium, potassium, zinc and some B Vitamins.

Walnuts The trees are native to the Far East. They are, however, grown in California, France, Spain, the USA and Italy. Best to buy them in a shell, they will keep fresher for longer that way. They help the digestion and improve metabolism. They are rich in calcium, iron, magnesium, zinc and Vitamin E.

There are plenty of other nuts to choose from - *macadamias* are large nuts from Australia. *Brazil nuts* come from the tropics, and have a three-sided shape. *Pecan nuts* are grown in the USA, and look similar to walnuts. *Pistachio nuts* are grown in the Near East and have a green color.

All edible nuts have healthful properties, as long as they are raw and unsalted.

Legumes or Pulses

Legumes, also known as *pulses*, include beans, peas, lentils and peanuts, and are the mature seeds that grow inside a pod. Legumes are nutritious, containing certain amino acids, vitamins and minerals plus plenty of fiber. They are a very important part of a vegetarian diet. Peanuts are also part of the legume family (although not recommended for regular consumption).

> *There are more than seventy different varieties of legumes. Beans are an important part of every known cuisine. They have been used for 10,000 years. In comparison, grains are the new kids on the block.*

Beans in general can help prevent cancer because they are high in fiber and low in fat and calories. Half a cup serving contains more than six grams of fiber plus potassium, zinc, iron and B Vitamins. Beans are a good source of protein though they do lack some essential amino acids. However, adding grains to the meal will provide the essential amino acids that are missing.

Studies have shown that the fiber in beans can lower blood cholesterol levels, reducing the risk of diabetes, heart attack and stroke.

Digestibility

·	Soya beans	- most difficult	*
·	Other beans in general	- fairly easy	**
·	Lentils	- easy	***
·	Sprouted beans and lentils	- very easy	****

Cooking Beans Correctly to Reduce Wind

Dried beans must first be soaked overnight, one part beans to four parts water. Afterwards, the water MUST be thrown away, as the gas-causing enzymes are released into the water while soaking them. Put the beans in plenty of fresh water, and while cooking add salt or a little seaweed, cumin seeds, fennel seeds or caraway seeds to make the beans even easier to digest. They must be brought to the boil and then boiled rapidly for twenty minutes without the lid on. Then cover with a lid and continue to simmer until soft. Cook large amounts and put the rest into the freezer, for when you are too busy.

If you still have trouble digesting beans, move to plan B. Look up sprouting.

The Most Common Pulses

Chickpeas support kidney function. They act as digestive cleansers and are a good source of calcium, magnesium, potassium, zinc, manganese, Vitamins B3, B5, B6 and folic acid. Chickpeas are used a lot in Middle Eastern and Indian cooking. The flour is known as gram flour.

Kidney beans are high in fiber, and cleanse the digestive tract. They increase beneficial bacteria and remove excess cholesterol. They are a good source of calcium, magnesium, phosphorus, potassium and folic acid.

Lentils, like other legumes, are a good source of soluble and insoluble fiber. Lentils are a good source of minerals for nearly every organ in the body. They neutralize acids produced in the muscles and provide calcium, magnesium and phosphorus. They are also a rich source of potassium, zinc, folic acid, plus loads of fiber.

Lentils help to lower cholesterol, but this is only one of many benefits derived from eating lentils. However, lentils, like most beans, are an incomplete protein, and for this reason, need to be eaten with whole grains to provide all the eight essential amino acids. They can be used in soups, stews or made into vegetarian pâtés, dips or dahl. Recipes for dahl can be found in Indian cookbooks. The whole lentils can also be sprouted. Lentils are found in different varieties - brown, green, very dark almost black and orange. However, the orange ones have had their skins removed and cannot be sprouted. Like beans, they are very cleansing.

Mung beans are small, round and green, a great heart and blood cleanser and excellent for detox. They are a good source of calcium, magnesium, iron, potassium, zinc, Vitamin B3, Vitamin B5 and folic acid. Easy to sprout.

Peanuts are not actually nuts, but legumes, and don't grow on trees or bushes like nuts. Peanuts actually grow in the ground, hence their other name, groundnuts. They grow like peas in a pod. The Spanish first stumbled across peanuts in South America; Now, China and India together produce more than fifty per cent of the world's peanuts. The US accounts for only five percent. Peanuts can slow down the metabolism of the liver, and should be avoided if you are overweight. If you can't put on weight, even though you eat a lot, add raw peanuts with their thin brown skins to your diet. Peanuts are heavily sprayed with agricultural chemicals.

Did You Know?
Americans eat enough peanut butter in a year to make ten billion sandwiches!

Soy beans are very hard to digest, which is why they are traditionally eaten in a fermented form, making them easier to digest. They are eaten in the form of tofu or soy sauce, tamari, tempeh, miso, etc (see below). Do not overdo it - eat soy products in moderation. Many of the world's soybeans have been genetically modified. Soybeans and soy products are rich in phyto-estrogens, hormone-like substances that mimic the action of estrogen in the body. In Japan, soybean products are very popular, and Japanese women rarely complain of menopausal problems. Studies have shown that women who eat foods rich in soy isoflavones and phyto-estrogens have lower rates of breast cancer than those who don't eat such foods. Even Japanese men who eat a lot of soy product have less prostate problems than their Western counterparts. What we must also bear in mind is that Japanese men and women eat far fewer refined and processed foods, more fresh produce, drink less alcohol, and smoke less - it isn't just down to eating fermented soy products. In general, their eating habits are far healthier than ours in the West. Health is never just down to one thing; nothing can be taken in isolation.

Tofu, also known as bean curd, is part of Oriental cuisine and is a really good source of protein. It has only four to five per cent fat, which is mainly unsaturated. The B Vitamins and minerals remain undamaged by the tofu-making process. It comes in two types: silken tofu, which can be used to replace cream in desserts and sauces, and the firm tofu, which has a soft, cheese-like consistency. Tofu can be used in sweet and savory dishes. There is one drawback (or benefit, depending on how you view it); tofu has no flavor at all. It's very bland, but this isn't a problem as it soaks up any flavor really easily. Tofu is made from dry soybeans, soaked and then crushed and boiled. A coagulant is added to this soymilk, which makes it separate into curds and whey, a similar process to cheese making. The curds are then poured into moulds and left to settle. Tofu's lack of taste makes it ideal for marinating. It's naturally low in fat and calories. Tofu can also be used as an alternative for cheesecakes.

Miso is a mixture made from fermented soy or barley with rice. It's a live food containing lactobacillus, aiding in digestion and assimilation. It also helps to create an alkaline environment in the body. Always get non-pasteurized miso, and it should only be added at the very last minute to cooked food, as cooking will destroy the live bacteria. Miso can be used instead of Worcestershire sauce, bouillon, stock cubes and soya sauce; it's a healthier option.

Soy sauce is made from wheat, soybeans, water and sea salt. Tamari, on the other hand, is a soy sauce made without wheat.

Tempeh is a soy product made via an enzyme process that creates a white fibrous mass, which is very nutritious. There are many varieties, made with a combination of soy with wheat, rice, peanuts or millet. It's easy to digest, high in protein and low in fat. Do not eat tempeh raw; it needs to be cooked really well.

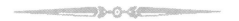

Chapter 15

Odds and Ends

"What is food to one man is bitter poison to others"
Lucretius

Thickeners

Here are some alternatives to white flour or white cornstarch for gravy
or sauces, etc.

Arrowroot is a powdered tropical root that is used as a thickener and is
   high in calcium. Often found in supermarkets where you would find
   baking powder or bicarbonate of soda.

Kuzu is a powdered tuber from Japan, used as a thickener that soothes
   the stomach and the intestines.

General

Here is a list of some health-giving alternatives to the staples of our
modern Western diet:

Agar-agar is used instead of gelatine, and is made from seaweed. It's a
   good source of calcium and iron. It contains no calories.

Gelatine is obtained from animal skins and bones, both by-products of
   slaughterhouses. Gelatine for the food industry is made mainly from
   pigskins or cattle-hides. You will find gelatine in jellies,
   confectionery, meat products and chilled dairy products like fromage
   frais. More gelatin is sold to the food industry than any other gelling
   agent. Gelatin for the pharmaceutical industry is made from cattle
   bones and is a more complex and costly process. Medicine capsules
   are made from this gelatin. In the health industry more and more
   supplements are now being produced using vegetable-based

capsules instead. These capsules tend to be a bit more expensive, but are worth it.

Apple cider vinegar Therapeutically, no other vinegar will do. Apple cider vinegar has a positive affect on the body's acid-alkaline balance. The organic acids are oxidized in the body, leaving an alkaline base residue in the blood. It's a rich source of alkaline-forming elements like potassium, calcium, magnesium, phosphorus, chlorine, sodium, sulfur, iron, fluorine, silicon, plus many trace minerals. This encourages a less acidic urine and blood. To improve digestion, take one to two teaspoons of apple cider vinegar in a little water thirty minutes before each meal. Researchers have found that the malic acid found in this vinegar helps to dissolve calcium deposits, therefore aiding in the relief of arthritis, rheumatism, kidney stones, etc.

Carob comes from the carob tree, native to the Mediterranean. The pod turns black when ripe and is then ground to a powder. Rich in natural sugar, calcium and minerals - use instead of sugar or chocolate in cooking or baking. It has less fat than cocoa powder and has not been roasted like cocoa.

Coconut milk isn't the liquid in the middle of the coconut. It's made by boiling ground coconut with water, forming a thick liquid that is then squeezed through a strainer. This is often used in Asian and Indian cooking.

Goat's milk Many people live with an undiagnosed cow's milk intolerance, with symptoms ranging from diarrhea, wind, bloating, stomach cramps and much more. These reactions are caused by a protein called alpha-S-1casein, found in cow's milk, but only found in tiny traces in goat's milk. Like human milk, goat's milk is composed mainly of beta-casein proteins, which are easier for most people to digest. Two cups of goat's milk will easily provide the minimum daily calcium requirement, where three cups of cow's milk barely do. Goat's milk exceeds cow's milk in short and medium-chain mono-unsaturated, polyunsaturated and essential fatty acids.

Lecithin is mainly derived from soybeans, although sometimes from egg yolks. It's a fatty substance that acts as an emulsifying agent. Lecithin enables fats, such as cholesterol and other lipids, to be dispersed in water and removed from the body. One or two dessertspoonsful of lecithin granules can be sprinkled on cereals, yogurts, soups, juices, etc. Lecithin also comes in capsules. Taking one capsule before meals helps the digestion of fats and absorption of fat-soluble vitamins. Lecithin is mainly composed of the B Vitamins choline and inositol, plus linoleic acid. Without lecithin, our cells would harden, as it protects our cells from oxidative damage. Other sources of lecithin are grains, legumes, fish and wheatgerm. Lecithin is also very important to the nervous system.

Natural Sweeteners

Here are some natural sweeteners that can be used as alternatives to white sugar - but they should still be used in moderation. You need to re-educate your taste buds to expect less sweet-tasting foods.

Dried fruit is a good substitute for sugar in recipes. Soak in water for a few hours first and then puree. Dates, apricots and figs are good for this, but any dried fruit can be used.

Fresh fruit, like mashed banana or grated apple, can be added to recipes to cut down on or avoid sugar. Add fresh fruit to natural 'live' yogurts.

Honey has been known for centuries for its healing properties. Cold pressed is really the best, as the enzymes haven't been destroyed in processing. Most honey is produced using high temperatures, destroying the enzymes. As we all know, honey is made from the nectar of flowers by bees. It has antibacterial properties (if cold pressed), and when used externally, it speeds up healing. Internally, it's very soothing and calming to the intestinal tract. It helps to maintain electrolyte balance, which is especially important during times of vomiting and diarrhea. Honey also enhances the healing properties of herbs, and is especially helpful for soothing the mucus lining of the respiratory system. Buy the best quality you can find or afford. Be careful not to consume too much of it, as it will interfere with your blood sugar levels in the same way ordinary sugar can, so use sparingly. Honey is made up of eighty per cent sugar and twenty per cent water, with only traces of minerals and enzymes, if it hasn't been heated in

> *It isn't safe to give honey to infants (up to about the age of twelve months), because it can contain spores of the bacterium C. botulinum. This isn't a problem to older children and adults, as normal stomach acid inhibits the growth of this bacterium.*

the manufacturing process. Locally produced fresh honey can be used to treat hay fever.

Muscovado sugar or molasses sugar is an unrefined, very dark brown sugar (the same color as black coffee). It retains all its nutrients.

Molasses syrup is thick and very, very dark brown. Two tablespoons contain almost as much calcium as a glass of milk, and it's also high in potassium and iron. Molasses is a by-product of the sugar refining industry. It's the syrup that remains after the sugar cane has been refined to produce white sugar. As we all know, white sugar is void of nutrients, so cooking and baking with molasses makes for a healthy alternative. It also contains chromium, which is vital for the health of the pancreas, enabling us to deal with sugar in the first place. The mineral chromium is removed in the white sugar refining process.

Maple syrup comes from wild-growing maple trees. It does contain a small amount of minerals, but use sparingly. It will still interfere with your blood sugar levels in the same way white sugar does. Make sure the maple syrup you buy is pure. Some have had refined sugar added to make the product cheaper. Read the label carefully.

Teas

Black tea Fermented leaves from the tea plant, containing caffeine and tannic acid. Tannic acid works like an astringent, drying up diarrhea. If you suffer from constipation, you need to consider giving up tea altogether. Tannic acid also hinders absorption of minerals, especially iron.

Mate tea A tea-like drink made from partially roasted holly leaves.

Rooibush tea (also known as rooibos, red bush tea and red tea) comes from a tall shrub in Africa. The leaves are fermented, and it contains no caffeine.

Green tea comes from the bush Camellia sinenis, which is widely cultivated in Asia, especially Japan. Green tea contains numerous anti-cancer compounds including catechin, a powerful antioxidant. It's low in caffeine, unlike black tea, and the taste is quite different. Green tea's many health benefits include: alleviating fluid retention; helping weight loss by increasing the metabolism of fat; regulating blood sugar and insulin levels; helping to lower cholesterol levels. Recent studies have shown that green tea may protect against certain cancers. To gain the benefits, drink the tea up to three times a day.

Avoid this tea if pregnant or nursing. The tea is sold in loose-leaf form or in tea bags, in varying qualities.

Herbal teas and fruit teas are so popular and come in such a wide variety of flavors that there are so many to choose from, too many to mention. Experiment, find some you enjoy drinking. Some health shops will sell individual tea bags, allowing you to try a bigger variety, without having to buy the whole box. These teas should be drunk without milk and sugar.

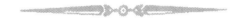

Chapter 16

In a Nutshell

We Need Hydrating Fluids

- to flush toxins out of our system
- to dilute urea
- to keep joints plump with plenty of fluid for cushioning
- to prevent muscles becoming stiff and painful
- to prevent constipation
- to maintain correct brain function.

We Need Enzymes

You may be wondering - if we make our own enzymes, why would we need to worry about consuming them? By just adding some enzymes to your diet you will be taking the load off your system, allowing your body to use its resources for other jobs. In other words, there are more resources left for regeneration.

We Need Co-enzymes (Vitamins and Minerals)

Vitamins and minerals are vital to the health of every cell, and we need to provide them with nutrient-rich food constantly. When we eat nutrient-poor foods, the body will have to rob nutrients from other functions to provide enough for digestion. The body can put off certain jobs until enough nutrients are provided, but digestion must be dealt with, come what may, even if it does it badly. Take, for example, white rice, which has had most of its B Vitamins removed. The body still needs Vitamin Bs to digest it. Brown rice provides B Vitamins for its digestion and there are some left over for other jobs within the body.

We Need Phyto-chemicals

There are too many phyto-chemicals to mention, and more are being discovered all the time. Phyto-chemicals are plant compounds that are vital to our health. For instance, ellagic acid, found in cherries, black grapes or strawberries, has powerful anti-cancer properties. There are hundreds of compounds that have a therapeutic effect, but unfortunately many people eat very little in the way of vegetables, fruits or herbs, so don't get the benefits of plant compounds.

We Need Fiber

There is something a little odd about the fact that we buy refined foods like white flour products that have had their nutrients removed or destroyed and all the fiber removed in processing. Then, at a premium price, we are sold some of the missing bits back. They sell us back the wheat bran, the wheat germ and finally nutrients in the form of tablets, separately. If you think about it, it's a very strange practice.

I come across a lot of people who add wheat bran to their highly refined diet.

1. It will not enhance your nutritional status.
2. If you are dehydrated, and most of us are, concentrated bran will make the situation worse.
3. Wheat bran is very concentrated and harsh, and for many people it can cause irritation to the delicate lining of the GI tract.
4. It can interfere with the absorption of iron and calcium.

I have nothing good to say about concentrated wheat bran, especially when we can get various types of fiber and nutrients easily from many whole foods available to us.

I don't want to give you the impression that I am against supplements of vitamins and minerals; far from it. But first and foremost, we need to build a good foundation with nutrients from natural whole foods - this is fundamental to our health. Supplements (vitamins, minerals, amino acids, etc), as the word implies, are additional or supporting.

It's important, however, to get some of this extra support if you:
· 	live in the city
· 	are an athlete
· 	are pregnant (check out with your doctor or naturopath)

·   are studying and taking exams
·   are experiencing extra stress
·   are menopausal
·   have a chronic problem
·   do heavy labor.

During these situations, a healthy diet plus some basic supplements would be a good idea.

To Recap

Look carefully at what you bring home from the supermarket. As the nation's diet declines, chronic diseases like arthritis, heart disease, diabetes, obesity and many more are on the increase.

·   Are you bringing home too many soft drinks, crisps, biscuits, white bread, processed packaged meals?
·   Are you bringing home enough fresh fruit and vegetables?
·   Are you drinking too much tea, coffee or alcohol?
·   If you smoke, how many?

Keep a Food Diary

As already suggested, try to keep a food diary, putting down everything you have been eating and drinking normally. Then study it. I think you will be surprised. The best way to change your diet is to do it gradually, so that it becomes a way of life. Start with the things you will find the easiest to change. This is especially important with children - change things gradually and slowly, so they don't notice it too much. However, we are all different and you may prefer to take the bull by the horns, by going for lots of changes straight away. That's fine too, but only if your body can cope.

You may want to look up a naturopath or nutritionist, getting support through your changes.

Study your Diary and Consider:

Your salt intake. You may not add salt to your food but there are many products that contain a lot of salt. For instance, cheese, crisps, Marmite, pre-made sauces, all delicatessen meats, processed meals, etc.

Your sugar intake. Cakes, biscuits, chocolates, jams, baked beans, soft drinks (which contain a lot of sugar). Don't be tempted to swap one poison for an even worse one. Don't be fooled by the claims of artificial sweeteners, and read the labels of low-fat products carefully, as you will be surprised where sugar crops up.

The amount of stimulants you take. Tea, coffee, cokes, chocolate, sugar, and alcohol should all find their way onto your hit list eventually.

Your fat intake from pastries, pies, cheese, butter/ margarine, cream, chocolate, cakes, biscuits and delicatessen meats. Be careful about using 'low-fat' products, as they can sometimes contain more sugar instead (which ultimately turns to fat).

Your fresh fruit and vegetable intake. The standard recommendation is five portions every day. This is the absolute minimum you should consume (not including potatoes). For good health you would ideally be eating more than the recommended minimum. What is a portion? One apple or one pear or one heaped handful of something like grapes or vegetables.

Your fiber intake. White bread, biscuits, pies, pastries, cakes, crisps and meats contain almost no fiber.

How often you fry food. Stir-frying should be considered as the best alternative to frying - especially if you use cold-pressed, virgin oils.

The amount of processed foods you eat. Processed foods contain additives, preservatives and anti-nutrients. All add to your toxic load, putting considerable strain on your eliminating organs.

How much water you drink. Water is vital for good health, so make sure you drink enough each day. Ideally you should be drinking six to eight glasses a day, but this would depend on your size, your activity levels and the weather. If you hate water, then drink herbal teas without milk or honey, or fruit juices diluted with fifty per cent water.

Your 'essential fatty acid' intake. These fatty acids, as the name suggests, are essential to us. They are found in foods like nuts and seeds (not roasted or salted).

How much live enzyme-rich foods you are eating. You should be eating plenty of the correct fruit, along with lightly cooked or raw vegetables, yogourt, etc.

Making Changes

Think about the areas of your diet where you think you can easily make changes, and do them first. Other changes may be easier than you think, if you try some alternatives to the food you are used to. Remember, it takes a little time to acquire a new taste, and to change the habits of a lifetime. The following chart will help you to plan a program of changes. Don't try changing more than a couple of items at a time; doing things gradually makes success much more attainable

Use this chart of alternatives to compose your shopping list.

CUT DOWN or AVOID	ALTERNATIVES
Pork and beef	Lamb (occasionally), chicken, duck, fish, tofu, or a combination of beans and grains
Cow's milk	Sheep, goat, rice, soy, oat or coconut milk
Chocolate	Carob, or very occasionally seventy per cent chocolate (it has far less sugar and processed fat)
Tea and coffee	Herbal/fruit teas, green tea, dandelion coffee, water
Cream	Natural live yogurt, silken tofu
Margarine	Extra virgin oil mixed with butter
Cow's cheese	Goat's and sheep's cheese
Couscous	Millet, quinoa, amaranth
Salt	More herbs and spices, 'low-sodium salt' or sea salt
Snacks	Dried / fresh fruit, homemade popcorn, nuts, seeds
Fizzy drinks	Fruit juices, diluted with carbonated water occasionally
White flour	Whole grain flours - millet, quinoa, brown rice, whole corn, buckwheat, barley, oat, amaranth, spelt, and kamut, rye, chickpea (gram) flour
Expensive processed, gluten-free products	Use millet, amaranth, quinoa, rice, corn, buckwheat. Avoid wheat, rye, barley, oats, spelt and kamut
White rice	Brown rice - there are many varieties
White sugar	Molasses, muscovado sugar, dried fruit soaked overnight and pureed
Thickeners for gravy, etc	Arrowroot or kuzu root for most things, or red lentils in soups
Oils	Any cold pressed or extra virgin oils (organic if possible)
Wheat bread	100% sourdough rye bread in moderation, rice/oat cakes, homemade breads from different grains
Breakfast cereals	Porridge, homemade muesli, puffed amaranth
Stock cubes	Miso, tamari, more herbs & spices, your own stock
White pasta	Japanese soba (spaghetti from buckwheat), rice noodles, a variety of pastas from various grains
Processed yogurts	Natural 'live' varieties

Most of us lead busy lives and don't want to spend every spare moment in the kitchen cooking. Make more use of your freezer. Invest in some large pots and always cook extra, for lunch the next day or for putting the rest in the freezer, for times when you are too busy to cook. Using your freezer isn't the perfect situation, fresh is always best, but it's always better than eating processed convenience foods from a factory, when you are in a hurry.

Some Kitchen Gadgets you May Want to Invest in

·   Juice extractor
·   Steamer (either for use on the stove top, or an electrical one)
·   Bread maker (simple and effortless to use)
·   Yogourt maker (makes the job simple)
·   Cast iron wok for stir fries
·   Popcorn maker for an instant snack for children (cheap to buy, very easy to use, hot air, no oil and the kids love using them)
·   Coffee grinder for seeds like linseeds, coriander, caraway, fennel, etc
·   Ice-cream maker for children
·   Blender
·   Sprouting gadget, or just some large glass jars with some netting and elastic bands

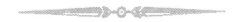

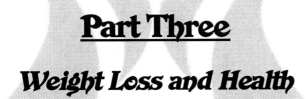

Part Three

Weight Loss and Health

Chapter 17

Dieting

"Now there are more overweight people in America than average weight people. So, overweight people are now average. Which means you've met your New Year's resolution"
Jay Leno

Let's take a look at obesity and some of the research done on fatty tissue. It was found that the fatty tissue of an overweight person was very deficient in lipase. Lipase, as we have already discussed, is the enzyme that aids in the breakdown of fat. There has been much research on this subject, and it has been discovered that eating dead food puts on weight. Dead food is void of enzymes and most often the necessary nutrients, which are used for burning fat for energy, storage and distribution. Without enough enzymes, our fat stagnates.

From my experience as a practitioner, I know some of you will be more convinced to change your way of eating if it's for weight reduction, rather than health risk reduction. The good news is you can achieve both, the naturopathic way.

What does the research evidence say about dieting and calorie counting?

- Over ninety-five per cent of dieters regain their original weight within two years, and many are left heavier than before; a depressing thought.
- After five years, ninety-eight per cent of dieters regain their weight! That's a lot of effort, and often much expense for little return.

We are starving our bodies, causing ourselves to become malnourished. Starvation of nutrients leads to overeating. It's nothing to do with will power; your body is crying out for nutrients. This can manifest itself as food cravings that can be as strong as an alcoholic's addiction.

The consequences of low-calorie dieting are food deprivation and starvation. The World Health Organization (WHO) states, through their experience with their worldwide starvation program, that starvation begins at less than 2,100 calories per day! It uses this as a basis for determining the organization's guidelines for emergency food aid. At 2,200 calories food aid packets comply with WHO standards, while many women in the West consistently eat a lot less.

·   Do you consistently eat less than 2,100 calories?
·   Do you skip meals?
·   Do you eat refined foods, empty calories?

Despite the fact that dieting has a mere two percent long-term success rate, we are dieting more often, more radically and from a younger age. Yet more people are overweight.

The body doesn't understand dieting; it understands starvation and famine. It must protect against any future famine. So as soon as the famine is over it must lay down reserves as quickly as possible before the next famine. This is an in-built survival mechanism.

Evidence has also shown that more than sixty per cent of dieters did not have a real weight problem before they started dieting. That was not the case after they had been on two or three diets.

Most dieters and even some non-dieters use diet drinks and diet foods to avoid calories. As discussed earlier, artificial sweeteners can contribute to compulsive eating. Several studies, in both animals and humans, show an increase in cravings for sweet and fatty foods.

We are now becoming 'low-carb' crazy. However, not all carbohydrates are created equal. Some will interfere with your blood sugar levels, encouraging insulin production and ultimately laying down fat, regardless of the amount of calories you consume. Certain other carbohydrates don't have this effect - they can have a positive effect on our health.

Not all fats are created equal, either. Some are essential to our health, as I mentioned in Part One, and even help to increase metabolism and prevent fluid retention to name but a couple of functions. Do you have a 'fat' or 'carbohydrate' phobia?

So, what is so different about a holistic approach?

Well, there is no such thing as calorie counting. It's what you eat and not how much you eat. There is no 'going on' and 'coming off' a diet. As statistics show time and time again, people don't maintain their weight loss over the years. Unlike the diet industry, a holistic approach doesn't use highly refined foods that contain many additives like artificial sweeteners. It certainly doesn't cause malnutrition, as proven to be the case for many dieters who don't eat enough of the right foods. Deficiencies will eventually set up cravings and cause chronic health problems. These chronic problems are on the increase, and there is a mountain of research to show that it's mainly due to our poor food choices. I have come across a lot of dieters who keep the diet food and drink industry very happy and wealthy by consuming loads of their artificial, processed foods and drinks, but still have a weight problem.

The holistic approach looks to redress cravings, food intolerance, deficiencies, fluid retention, cellulite and detoxing by changing your eating habits forever. You need to feed your body, not starve it. You will be able to make informed choices that will affect you for the rest of your life. Every day more and more evidence is being produced to show that our eating habits are contributing to our weight problems.

Many people are in a trap and have no idea how to get out of it. We now know, from experience and the evidence, that dieting in the long run leaves us in worse shape than before we started dieting in the first place. When I say in worse shape, our bodies can change shape by losing muscle and regaining fat but also our health is left in worse shape. In the West, the fact is a lot of us are eating fewer calories and getting fatter! How do we escape? This is where we look closely at health issues to help sort out our weight problems.

I often hear people say, 'If I had more willpower I wouldn't have come off my diet, I would have stuck with it.' It's not a matter of willpower. I see people who have plenty of willpower and discipline in every aspect of their lives, often losing loads of weight over and over again.

As I have already suggested, keep a food diary, and write down everything you eat and drink normally. Even if you read on, at this point don't change your diet yet. Wait seven days until you have finished your diary, including your symptoms like headaches, moods, tiredness, etc. If you are only interested in weight loss, and have turned straight to this section, I suggest you go back and read the first two parts of this book, as you will gain a far better understanding of how your body interacts with the foods you consume.

Weigh yourself occasionally, but not daily. Instead, measure your hips, bust, upper arms, thighs, waist and knees. Keep a record of these measurements to refer to in the months to come.

I need to warn you that this isn't a quick-fix solution. Changing the habits of a lifetime will take a few weeks or months but then you will be free. Free from addiction, low-energy bingeing, yo-yo weight loss and gain, problematic periods, headaches, bad skin, emotional problems, constipation and much more. Once you change your habits, you will automatically want to follow a healthier way of life, because you will feel so much better and be slimmer.

The main points we need to address are:
1. Low-calorie dieting will have left you malnourished and deficient.
2. Stabilizing 'blood sugar levels' - which can set up food cravings, moodiness, anxiety and headaches.
3. Adrenal and thyroid function.
4. Detoxing.
5. Brain chemistry.
6. Yeast overgrowth and a leaky gut, mentioned earlier in this book.

Have you ever been on a diet? Some people answer that they feel as if they have been on a diet nearly all their lives. Do you ever skip meals? Do you eat less than 2,100 calories a day? Currently, in Britain, nearly seventy per cent of fifteen year olds are dieting! In the US back in 1964, fifteen per cent of people were dieting, yet in 1992, seventy per cent of women, fifty per cent of men and eighty per cent of teenagers were dieters. Today, even nine-year-old children are dieting! Yet for all of this dieting, we are generally getting fatter. Clearly, something needs to be done.

Low calorie dieting just adds up to starvation. The body doesn't understand today's vogue of skinniness; it only understands survival. Prisoners in concentration camps were fed 900 calories a day. I know people who eat that or not much more than that. They may well find the World Health Organization has left a food aid parcel on their doorstep!

The consequences of low-calorie dieting are:
- Loss of self-esteem
- Forty per cent drop in metabolic rate
- Muscle shrinkage
- Decrease in heart output by forty per cent
- Return to pre-diet weight
- Preoccupation with food
- Gallstones, and sometimes the removal of the gall bladder due to low-calorie dieting and liquid diets (twenty-five per cent of liquid dieters develop gallstones and need their gall bladder removed).
- Mental dullness
- Increased risk of developing diabetes
- Decreased sexual interest
- Elevated cholesterol levels
- Elevated uric acid levels
- Nausea
- Headaches
- Abnormal heartbeat
- Mood swings
- Binging and cravings

It's a shame that we are more preoccupied with our superficial look than our internal health. I find that people will not eat more fruit and vegetables to prevent cancer or stave off chronic diseases, but are happy to eat nasty chemicals in the hope of losing weight. With the promise of the latest diet delivering a miracle, people will follow some very strange eating plans that can put their health at serious risk, and are often more than happy to use drugs, laxatives, stimulants and diuretics. Yet many people are not prepared to put themselves out much for the sake of their health. But our health is the most precious thing we could have. If you say to someone, 'I can't eat that, as I'm on a diet and am starving myself,' that's fine. Yet, if you say to someone, 'I don't eat this or that because it's not healthy,' the reaction is quite different.

When animals are put through a number of restricted-calorie diets, after a while they begin to show a greater preference for fatty foods, compared to animals that have never been on a diet. This seems to be the same for us also. An article in the New England Journal of Medicine reported the findings of a researcher who analyzed the records of the famous Framingham Heart Study. It concluded that those who had a fluctuating weight had a seventy-five per cent greater risk of heart disease.

> ### How to Fatten a Pig for Market
> *The farmer restricts the amount of food the animal is allowed for several days, then for a few days, the animal is allowed to eat as before. Farmers have found these animals go to market heavier than those who have been fed constantly.*

Metabolic Rate

One way that dieting causes us to store more fat is through lowering our metabolic rate. During a restricted diet, metabolism can be reduced by as much as forty per cent. Metabolism is the process of using energy for a whole host of functions within the body. Those of us who diet, dramatically decrease the number of calories that are metabolized during exercise, and even during normal activities throughout the day. It only takes a couple of days for the body to switch the metabolic rate to a lower setting. Research shows that women who are restrained eaters eat on average 410 fewer calories per day than non-dieters, but burn fewer calories per day than those who are non-dieters. It doesn't seem fair. Each diet lowers the metabolic rate more than the previous diet and it takes longer each time for the metabolic rate to recover. I often hear people complain that their present diet isn't working as well as the last few times.

An article written by Dr Allen King, called 'Obesity and Health', demonstrated how he put 500 of his patients on a 1,000-calorie-a-day diet. Six months later, the average patient had lost fifty pounds - success, you would think. After three years, these same patients had gained an average of sixty pounds - depressing! For some, it didn't take as long as three years.

Other research shows that a restricted diet seems to reduce the activity of the thyroid gland by about twenty-eight per cent in only six weeks. Similar reductions have been noted in animals on a restricted diet.

Fat Storage

An enzyme called adipose tissue lipoprotein lipase (LPL) helps the body to store fat for the lean times. Transport of fat from the blood to the fat cells depends on this enzyme. In people who have restricted their calories to lose weight, the activity of LPL is much increased.

The very action of dieting greatly increases the activity of this potent, fat-storing enzyme. Once you start eating again (which you will do eventually, as you cannot starve yourself forever) you will regain all you have lost, plus a little extra just for good measure.

LPL and Insulin

Insulin stimulates the quantity and activity of LPL, which seems to be the prime method by which it fattens. Much more about this later, as it's a very important aspect to the whole health/weight plan.

Insulin is also adept at slowing metabolic rate. Dieting may also induce changes in the action of an enzyme known as sodium-potassium ATP-ase. This is a fat-burning enzyme, which is significantly lower in dieters. Dieting may therefore increase our fat-storing enzymes while lowering fat-burning enzymes. Not ideal for losing weight.

It makes sense as our bodies are set for survival (during famine) - it's the law of nature, our bodies are not set for a photo shoot with Vogue magazine.

Genes

Genes can make a difference, but they are by no means the whole picture. You may have inherited a tendency to be overweight, but you don't have to make it your plight. You can offset this weakness with the right lifestyle or you can encourage this weakness with the wrong sort of diet. We must not overlook the fact that bad habits are learnt/inherited and taste buds are developed from childhood, depending on what our parents fed us.

In just about every case of a traditional society moving to towns and cities and adopting a more 'Western-type diet', they start to suffer all the things we do. For instance, American Indians or the Australian Aboriginals were formerly lean and suffered very little diabetes. Now they have high rates of obesity and suffer chronic problems at similar rates to us. This isn't entirely due to genes, but due to a change in lifestyle. At the turn of the last century in the US about five per cent of people were overweight. Now it's estimated that about sixty-five per cent of Americans are overweight. This isn't a genetic problem; it's due to a change in our eating habits and lifestyles.

Food Addiction

One third to about half of people on a diet eat compulsively, having developed food cravings, and for some these cravings can be as strong as alcohol, drug or nicotine addiction. Most people have had these food cravings since childhood; they just didn't realize it. For others the cravings began after a diet or two. Your body can fight back against starvation by escalating food cravings until they are strong enough to overwhelm the will to diet, and for some these cravings don't go after they have stopped dieting and regained the weight.

As you crave and devour refined carbohydrates, these 'drug foods' can create a false high in the brain. Some people then overeat, consuming loads of empty calories through white sugar and white flour. This leaves them malnourished, as these foods will use up valuable resources, depleting the body's reserves. These are what we call empty calories. They will leave you wanting more.

Which foods do you love? Which foods do you think you would be unable to live without? These could very well be the foods you are addicted to. You have been using these foods like a drug and will need to eliminate them from your diet altogether, just like the alcoholic who isn't able to have even one small drink.

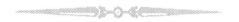

Chapter 18

The Food Industry

"As I see it, every day, you do one of two things: build health or produce disease in yourself"
Adelle Davis

The food industry is well aware that people crave wheat, sugar, salt and dairy products. They have made full use of this fact - everywhere you look there are products made from wheat, processed fats, sugar and far more salt than necessary. This is why natural foods can taste bland, but it doesn't take long for you to acquire a taste for them. You can add plenty of health-promoting herbs and spices to enhance their taste.

Coffee and Caffeine

Caffeine is found in coffee, teas, soft drinks like cokes, some painkillers, some energy drinks, and some slimming products. Read labels carefully.

Coffee gives you a lift, helps you to get out of bed in the morning - it even helps some people cope with their day. The rich aroma and flavor are so inviting. So, what's wrong with coffee? Well, several things, like mineral depletion, exhausted adrenal glands, indigestion, anxiety and heart disease!

To 'just quit' is very much easier said than done, as there are those nasty caffeine withdrawal headaches and energy lows. And another horrible thought, what are you going to drink instead? Coffee addicts expect their drink to give them the jolt that caffeine is renowned for. But does coffee really give you that energy boost? Caffeine contains no calories so it doesn't provide energy. In fact, coffee does quite the opposite - it drains our energy and increases our stress levels. You may decide to stop reading at this point, thinking to yourself, that can't be true. But read on. What caffeine actually does is stimulate the adrenal glands to produce the hormones involved in the 'fight and flight' response. So what actually happens when we keep our bodies in a constant state of emergency by stimulating them with caffeine?

Genetic factors and your lifestyle determine how long you can continue to make repeated demands on your reserves and still maintain good health. Are you one of those coffee or tea drinkers who have no trouble sleeping after a shot of caffeine? You need to ask yourself, why have your adrenal glands stopped responding? What does that say about the health of your adrenal glands? The adrenal glands produce more than 150 hormones, including DHEA, testosterone, estrogen and cortisol. Caffeine has been shown in numerous clinical trials to elevate the blood's levels of cortisol, which in turn can compromise the immune system and interfere with the body's ability to fight infection. It also lowers the brain's stress threshold.

Caffeine can result in the following health problems:
· Blood sugar problems, caused by forcing the liver to release glycogen into the bloodstream, which in turn causes the pancreas to secrete excess insulin, producing a sharp drop in blood sugar (hypoglycemia). This can set up hunger and cravings in some people.
· Acid/alkaline imbalance. More than 208 acids in coffee contribute to indigestion and a variety of health problems caused by over-acidity.
· Mineral depletion. Caffeine forces the body to excrete calcium, potassium, iron and trace minerals - all essential to good health. This can lead to cravings for certain foods in the search to replace these lost nutrients.
· For pregnant women, caffeine crosses the placenta to the fetus, and studies indicate a higher incidence of miscarriage, infertility and low infant birth weight.
· Pre Menstrual Tension/Syndrome and fibrocystic breast disease are both aggravated by caffeine. As we all know PMS can cause some of us to crave or binge on certain foods. Never fruit and vegetables - usually chocolate, crisps or biscuits.
· It worsens hot flushes and other symptoms caused by hormonal imbalances.
· Men with prostate problems should be aware that coffee irritates the urinary tract and bladder. Eliminating caffeine often relieves

symptoms associated with frequent urination due to an enlarged prostate gland.

·   It's a diuretic, which is dehydrating.

I can hear you saying, what about decaf? Decaffeinated coffee still contains 7mg of caffeine per cup, enough to get healthy adrenal glands kick-started. More importantly, decaf also contains all the coffee acids and harsh oils that can cause liver and digestive problems. In fact, the process of producing a decaf coffee removes some of its flavor, so a more strongly flavored Robusta bean is used, which tends to be more caustic than the usual Arabica bean. The acids in any coffee put a strain on the body's acid/alkaline balance. In order to neutralize these acids, our bodies use calcium as a buffering agent. Coffee depletes calcium, increasing the risk of osteoporosis.

Coming Off Caffeine

Caffeine withdrawal headaches often come with fatigue. Caffeine constricts blood vessels in the brain and decreases circulation. Without caffeine the sudden increased circulation causes headaches. Be kind to your adrenal glands. Here are some tips to avoid those headaches and feeling so tired.

Plan to come off caffeine over a period of seven to fourteen days, depending on how much caffeine you consume. You can do this by drinking one cup of coffee less every day.

Start introducing herbal teas or coffee substitutes such as:

Roasted barley - high in potassium and iron, it reduces acid in the digestive tract. Also called 'Barley Cup', it has a deep nutty flavor.

Roasted carob - a nutritious sweet food, often used as a chocolate substitute - high in calcium and Vitamin A.

Roasted chicory root - high in potassium and calcium. Chicory helps digestion and lowers acidity. The French often add chicory to their coffee to help counteract its effects.

Roasted dandelion root coffee - high in potassium, helps the liver.

The above coffee substitutes can be added to your coffee in increasing amounts to wean yourself off coffee gradually.

Potassium is an electrolyte that stimulates nerve impulses, helps oxygenate the brain and enhances athletic performance.

Just a quick word to all you tea drinkers - it also contains caffeine and has its own set of problems too. Tea is a rich source of tannic acid, which hinders the absorption of minerals, especially iron. Tannic acid is a powerful astringent, which is very drying.

Refined Carbohydrates

Most people eat refined carbohydrates that have had their nutrients and fiber removed. This includes foods like biscuits, cakes, pastries, pasta, cereals and other foods made of white flour, processed refined fats and white sugar. These foods can trigger powerful brain chemicals to be released. People often say these foods energize, comfort or relax them. As time goes on it takes more of these carbohydrates to deliver the drug-like effect, eventually leading to stronger cravings and for some it can mean bigger binges.

Rates of diabetes have risen parallel to weight gain, over the past twenty years. In the past ten to twenty years our consumption of fat has dropped, while our consumption of refined carbohydrates and sugar has risen.

The average person eats more than 45kg/100lbs of sugar every year! This is just an average figure; some of you will be consuming much more. Check your food diary, you may be surprised. Back in 1900, the average American and Briton ate 11kg/25lbs of sugar a year - what a difference.

Refined carbohydrates can rapidly increase our insulin levels, causing considerable stress on our pancreas and adrenal glands. These foods deplete our vitamin and mineral reserves, the very nutrients that protect us from cravings and overeating. According to Professor Stephen O'Rahilly of Cambridge University, in the British Journal of Medicine, diabetes is the fastest-growing disease in the world. If you change your habits of a lifetime, you will cut your chances of getting this awful disease. The choice is yours.

Artificial Sweeteners

A lot of people have turned to these artificial chemicals to consume less sugar and hence less calories. Artificial sweeteners contribute to compulsive eating for some users. Several studies have revealed the very ironic fact, in both human and animal trials, that these sweeteners set up cravings for sweet and fatty foods. These effects are amplified when taken with caffeine (tea, coffee, coke, even decaf contains some caffeine). Artificial sweeteners have also been found to increase appetite! Besides being toxic, they can be very addictive and harder to give up than you think. For more information, look up "artificial sweeteners" in the index at the back of this book.

Sugar

Sugar may be legal and cheap, but it's very destructive. Our biochemical imbalances are far more powerful than our willpower.

It's a monster problem that demands you keep feeding it with refined carbohydrates and sugar.

Many symptoms of hypoglycemia (low blood sugar) are similar to adrenal exhaustion. When our blood sugar levels drop because of poor food choices, or by dieting or skipping meals, the adrenal glands produce and release adrenaline, which can make you nervous, jittery and irritable. It's hard work for the adrenals each time they have to perform this emergency procedure. If you are a dieter, your blood sugar levels will be low. Dieting and too much exercising can put a huge strain on the adrenal glands. There is no greater stress than impending death, which is what the adrenal glands perceive when we restrict calories. Remember our systems are set up to preserve the body in every way possible during times of famine.

Sugar can cause side effects like joint pain, headaches and hyperactivity. It works very much like alcohol would on our systems! It can cause mood and energy swings, hangovers, headaches, agitation and irritability. Sugar is very acid forming, as we all know it has the ability to rot teeth. Sugar of any type is able to hinder the white blood cells' ability to ingest pathogens for up to four or five hours after its ingestion. What is this doing to our immune systems? It's vitally important if you or any member of you family is suffering an infection to strictly avoid sugar of any type. These problems are only the tip of the iceberg.

Alcohol is a super sugar and very stressful to the adrenal glands.

Cigarettes - this will come as a surprise, but cigarettes are heavily laced with sugar. The cigarette industry is one of the biggest consumers of sugar. I too was surprised when I first discovered this fact.

As well as having sugar cravings, do you have salt cravings? If you do, you can be sure your adrenals are struggling. This leaves them less able to help you cope with illness, trauma and the daily stresses of life.

The following list will help you to keep track of where sugar lurks, ,under the many impressive sounding names it is given nowadays.

Sugar comes in many guises. You will need to read labels carefully.
   Look out for words ending in -ose and -ol:
· Dextrose
· Fructose
· Galactose
· Glucose
· Lactose
· Levulose
· Maltose
· Sucrose
· Mannitol
· Sorbitol
· Xylitol
· Corn syrup
· Maltodextrins

Sugar Censorship
Sugar is like a drug. When sugar was first introduced to Europe in the sixteenth century, it was kept under lock and key, as they recognized how addictive it was. It was worth its weight in silver.

Chapter 19

Blood Sugar

Junk carbohydrates and sugars are highly addictive - sadly, some of you will know only too well. You may have given these foods up for a short while during a 'diet' but find yourself going back to them time after time.

Our bodies and brains are constructed from protein, water, fat, vitamins and minerals. Our bodies can't use carbohydrates for building body structures; they are used as fuel. Carbohydrates are like the petrol in our cars - they are used for energy but can't be used as part of the construction. Our bodies need good quality fuel to function properly, not just any type of carbohydrate. Our cars also need the right type of fuel to function well.

If you are a carbohydrate junkie, and many dieters are, then you are constantly running on low. Paradoxically, you could be eating more refined carbohydrates and sugar yet your blood sugar levels are still continually running low. Like any addiction, we end up needing more and more over time to have the same affect. As you eat all these sweets, chocolates and refined starches, they enter the bloodstream very quickly, overwhelming and shocking our systems. The body needs to respond to bring high blood sugar levels down by producing insulin. Insulin's job is to lower blood sugar levels when they get too high, and it ultimately stores this excess as body fat!

As time goes on, you start to store this excess fatty weight from consuming too many refined carbohydrates. So the more refined carbohydrates you eat the more insulin you need. Insulin does its job rather too well, as it removes too much glucose from our bloodstream, causing 'low blood sugar' levels. At this point, most of you will go for something that will raise your blood sugar levels again. Now you have set up a vicious circle that isn't that easy to break.

Chronic low blood sugar is also known as hypoglycemia, which can cause you to be irritable, headachy, or unable to concentrate until you have eaten refined carbohydrates and/or sweets. From now on, keeping your blood sugar levels stable is a priority. You will then be able to eliminate highly addictive foods that contain sugar and white flour, which have no nutritional value, robbing your body of nutrients.

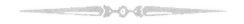

Chapter 20

Hormones

"Bad men live that they may eat and drink, whereas good men eat and drink that they may live"
Socrates (469 BC - 399 BC

Some of our worst cravings happen pre-menstrually and pre-menopausally. These can be very powerful indeed. Changes in diet, herbs and supplements will help to calm your brain chemistry and balance hormones. Estrogen stimulates the production of serotonin (our natural Prozac), as well as norepinephrine (our natural caffeine) and endorphins (our natural painkiller). For some women, estrogen levels drop too low, and hence PMS and menopause problems occur. So, as the levels drop, hormonal food cravings are magnified. From the age of about thirty-five, our ovaries begin to slow their production of estrogen, and eventually the adrenal glands need to start producing hormones to compensate. We need to be kind to our adrenal glands, but unfortunately, for many years, most of us have abused them.

In more traditional societies where women eat more healthily, they tend to suffer far less PMS or menopausal symptoms. In poorer countries, people tend to eat nutrition-rich foods, and little in the way of fast foods, processed or refined foods.

How have we upset our hormones over the years?
· not eating plenty of vegetables and fruit
· not getting enough protein
· not eating a healthy breakfast
· not giving up smoking
· not getting enough fiber

· not getting enough nutrients
· not giving up caffeine
· not getting enough hydrating fluids.

Alcohol and 'drug foods' (chocolate, sugar, refined carbohydrates) can alter our hormonal balance by impairing our liver function. Plus, the above foods rob our bodies of nutrients, often the very nutrients needed to produce adequate hormones, leaving us deficient in so many ways.

Chemical hormones are found in meat, poultry, milk, and now in farmed fish. These animals can be fed estrogen-like drugs to fatten them up for market. Plastic packaging contains chemicals from the petrochemical industry that mimic estrogen. So much food and drink today comes in plastic containers or wrapping, even water, and these chemicals can leach out into our food and water.

Adrenal Glands

Enter the two little adrenal glands, rushing to the rescue - they are the emergency team. The adrenal glands produce hormones to make sure your blood sugar levels don't drop too low, forcing the liver to get involved. As you can see, while you make poor food choices, your system is put under a lot of unnecessary stress.

Sooner or later, your adrenal glands will suffer. This is especially so if you lead a stressful life, drink too much caffeine and are short of nutrients. As you start to feel worse, you will end up consuming drug-like foods and drinks more often. This state of hypoglycemia is common amongst women, but is also experienced by men.

Some symptoms of adrenal exhaustion:
· sensitivity to fumes
· mood swings
· dark circles under the eyes
· dizziness on standing up a little too quickly
· lack of alertness
· tendency to catch a cold easily during the change of seasons
· headaches
· salt cravings
· sleep disturbances
· tired after a night's sleep
· feeling stressed

- need for caffeine to get you going in the morning
- startle easily
- food intolerance
- recurrent chronic infections, such as yeast types
- low tolerance to alcohol
- sensitivity to bright light
- feeling weak
- chronic heartburn or other digestive problems
- lack of thirst
- sweet craving
- alternating constipation and diarrhea
- nervousness
- exhaustion
- depression
- forgetfulness
- anxiety
- rapid pulse
- muscle aches
- crying spells
- leg cramps
- blurred vision.

Our adrenal glands help us to deal with all sorts of stress. They also help the thyroid to regulate our weight.

Here are some things that affect our adrenal glands negatively:
- going hungry
- skipping meals
- fasting
- eating too many refined foods
- eating too much salt
- sugar
- overworking
- drinking caffeine
- too much alcohol
- too much stress
- not getting enough sleep.

Thyroid

For some people, dieting can cause an already sluggish thyroid gland to become even more sluggish. The thyroid is a butterfly-shaped gland situated in the throat, under your Adam's apple.

All the glands work in partnership with other glands to maintain a hormonal balance throughout the body. None of them work in isolation.

Low-calorie dieting and nutritional deficiencies can affect the functions of the thyroid. Within hours of starting a restricted-calorie diet, the thyroid will slow down.

What can affect the thyroid?

· pregnancy
· puberty and dieting at the same time (more common these days, as more and more children are dieting earlier, some as young as nine years old).
· miscarriage
· removal of the ovaries
· menopause
· being short of iodine
· eating too many soy products, as they can inhibit the production of the primary hormone T4. In the Orient, some soy is eaten in the form of tofu, tempeh, etc. In the West the popular press jumped on the bandwagon, declaring soy good for us and suddenly soy was found in thousands of different products. Soy is extremely hard to digest, which is why it's most often fermented first for easier digestion.
· physical injury, such as whiplash
· severe illness
· chemicals in water, such as chlorine or fluoride
· some pharmaceutical drugs
· nutritional deficiencies.

If you suspect you have a problem with your thyroid, it might be worth making an appointment with a naturopath, herbalist, etc. A simple test and a case study will reveal what sort of program you should be on.

If your thyroid gland does turn out to be a little sluggish, it wouldn't necessarily show up on a conventional test. It would be treated by a change in diet, some supplements and herbs, which would help to balance the other glands that also affect the thyroid. But if it were discovered that your thyroid function is more than slightly sluggish, your next step would be to see your doctor. You may have to go on Thyroxin for the rest of your life.

How did you Become Addicted?

It might have been too many refined carbohydrates and sweets as a child, too many diets in the past, or nutritional deficiencies, yeast overgrowth, too much stress or any combination of these.

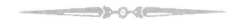

Chapter 21

Yeast Infections

"Tell me what you eat, and I will tell you what you are"
Anthelme Brillat-Savarin (1755-1826): The Physiology of Taste, 1825

Could Yeast be your Problem?

There is a lot of skepticism in the medical community about just how common yeast infections are. For some people it's a very real problem. There are many different types of yeast commonly found in the body and the air. From the time we are born we have yeast living in our intestines. Normally, this yeast lives in harmony with us. However, given the right set of circumstances, this yeast can overgrow in our bodies and cause a problem, often called a 'yeast infection', 'fungal infection' or 'candida'. When this infection shows up in the vagina or mouth it's called 'thrush', but can show up in other places. Researchers have estimated that about a third of us suffer from a yeast or fungal condition. This could be the cause of your food cravings, especially for refined carbohydrates and sugar.

How and why we get this problem

·   The use of antibiotics, wonderful as they are, will kill the 'good guys' as well as the 'bad guys'. As the 'friendly guys' are killed off by antibiotics, they allow some of the 'unfriendly guys' to take over.
·   The hormones in the contraceptive pill can encourage yeast overgrowth.
·   Spermicidal creams and foams contain Nonoxynol 9, which can destroy the vagina's friendly environment.
·   Cortisone and similar steroids can encourage yeast growth as these medications suppress the immune system.

- Refined carbohydrates and sugar - yeast loves these sorts of food.
- Poor digestion, i.e. low levels of hydrochloric acid, could be a problem. The correct levels will inactivate yeast.
- Nutritional deficiencies.
- Prolonged stress can weaken the immune system.
- Alcohol and tobacco can stress the liver, adrenal glands and immune system.

The more you feed the yeast with sugars, refined carbohydrates and alcohol, the more it reproduces and releases toxins.

Here are some symptoms (this list is by no means comprehensive):
- mental fog
- mood swings
- lethargy
- headaches
- sweet cravings
- susceptibility to infection
- sensitivity to pollutants
- achy joints and muscles
- dislike of damp weather or damp places.

These can also be symptoms of other things, and not necessarily a yeast infection.

Chapter 22

Fats

"I went into a McDonald's yesterday and said, 'I'd like some fries.'
The girl at the counter said, 'Would you like some fries with that?"
Jay Leno

We have become a fat-phobic society as the popular press has bombarded us with confusion and misinformation. We have thrown out the baby with the bath water, as the saying goes, and in doing so, many people have become addicted to fat. Ironic. We view all fats as the enemy. Our recent 'low-fat' mania has been causing health problems, causing us to become 'essential fatty acid' deficient.

Do you crave foods like chocolate, crisps, ice-cream, cream sauces and cheese or bread with lots of butter? If this is the case, then you are eating too many of the wrong fats and will be deficient in the right fats!

Where weight is concerned, some fats and oils can be stored in the body as an excess, not just on hips but more dangerously in our arteries and around our organs. However, other fats and oils can help us burn off calories and help keep our arteries and organs clear! It has been estimated that most of us only get about a tenth of the type of fats we need. The right dietary fat controls how much fat our bodies burn, and how fast it's burnt. If you are on a 'low-fat' diet regimen, you may very well end up rebounding and start over eating fats again as soon as you 'come off' the diet. Many find themselves gaining weight and becoming one of those statistics.

These fats are called 'essential fatty acids', and as you would imagine, they are essential to our well-being. 'Essential' means we cannot manufacture them for ourselves, so we need a constant supply from our diet. These good fats are needed for the production of hormones, they protect our internal organs, they keep our skin supple, and help maintain mental stability and concentration. They are very important to our metabolism and balancing our fluid levels. These fats help us to treat carbohydrate cravings, help to keep our bowels regular, to make and absorb certain fat-soluble vitamins like Vitamins A and E, protect against heart disease, inflammation, etc. The exact amount of fat isn't as important as the type of fat you eat.

We need to get enough Omega-3 'fatty acids' from foods like fish, leafy greens, nuts like fresh walnuts and linseeds, plus fatty acids from foods like butter and coconut. By consuming the correct fats you will begin to turn off your fat cravings, and you will also make it easier to eliminate your other cravings.

Most of us get enough Omega-6, but are short of Omega-3. In the West, the ratio is 20:1 when it should be about 2:1! This is a big difference. We are getting far too much Omega-6 and far too little Omega-3. The whole story of fats has been distorted in the past and is now causing health problems. Omega-3 fatty acids, when taken in the correct balance, will raise our metabolic rate and help us to lose weight as we burn calories more efficiently. Omega-3 also acts as a natural diuretic, helping the kidneys to flush excess fluids from our tissues, without causing them stress.

Prior to 1910, people ate diets high in fats and the rate of heart disease and obesity was much lower. The 1950s and 1960s gave us The Beatles, the mini skirt and cholesterol hysteria. We have thrown out all natural fats like butter, nuts, seeds, avocados, coconuts, and other tropical oils and fats from meats, in favor of highly processed fats and refined oils. Enter the silent killers that are contributing to some of our most common chronic conditions. Nearly all the oils and fats found on the supermarket shelves are highly processed and are very rancid, not that you would know it, as one of the many processes is to deodorize the oil so you can not taste or smell this.

Fixing your Fat Craving

You need to stop those fat cravings by giving your brain and your body the fats they need and removing the junk fats. The junk fats, like margarine and most oils found on the supermarket shelves are as refined and processed as white flour or white sugar and every bit as destructive.

Remember: 'essential fatty acids' promote weight loss.

Cholesterol

'Cholesterol' is a word most people consider equal to 'poison'. Yet it's much closer to the truth that processed oils are poisons. Cholesterol is so important that if we don't consume any, our body will just make more! Yes, our bodies make their own cholesterol. Our hormones depend on cholesterol so much that our bodies will make their own if we don't supply enough. Every cell in our bodies depends on cholesterol. Most of us don't have a problem with cholesterol as the body has some very good strategies in place for disposing of any excesses of this natural fat. However, the processed oils are so new and foreign to the body's processing mechanisms it has real difficulty dealing with them. There is just a small percentage of people who make too much cholesterol.

Generally, thirty per cent of the cholesterol we need comes from our diet, and the liver makes the rest. So, if you decide not to consume any cholesterol the body will just make more. It has been found in autopsies that processed oils account for seventy-four per cent of the build-up of plaque in our arteries. In our rush to throw out natural fats we have ended up eating too much toxic fat. These apparently healthy vegetable oils are hydrogenated, a process that turns liquid oils into more solid fats at room temperature - this is what we call margarine. The result is something called 'trans fatty acids' that are very damaging indeed. The body has not evolved to handle such molecules, which are used extensively in the food industry. For the sake of your health and your weight, you need to avoid processed fats altogether.

Have you been eating a low-fat diet, only to find yourself eating too many refined carbohydrates instead? This is a common problem. We need a certain amount of fat, but it must be the right type to turn off hunger and trigger a satisfaction sensation. The 'low-fat' highly refined carbohydrates will turn to fat, leaving you feeling hungry and wanting more. This fact has been known for years.

Fat Digestion: How is Yours?

Any foods we eat need breaking down fully so we can absorb and utilize their nutrients properly. So you could be eating the right sorts of fats, but not be getting their full benefit. You need enough enzymes and your liver and gall bladder need to be performing well. You may even have had your gall bladder removed.

Symptoms of digesting fats poorly include:
· Feeling overly full or heavy
· Feeling slightly nauseous
· Burping and belching after eating fatty foods
· Bloating
· Discomfort on the right upper side
· Indigestion
· Pain.

There are two very important requirements for fat digestion and utilization - bile and the enzyme lipase. Bile emulsifies fat, meaning it breaks it down into smaller droplets to increase the surface area so that the enzyme lipase can do its job properly. Bile is made by the liver and stored in the gall bladder. In the short term, it may be necessary at first to take supplements of digestive enzymes, which include lipase (found in health shops).

Once you have improved your eating habits, and hence your health, over the next few months, digestion will improve along with absorption. The pancreas will get the nutrients and proteins it needs to produce enough digestive enzymes. The body will no longer be stressed by a high-carbohydrate diet. Liver and gall bladder function will improve and the body will no longer be working overtime to produce insulin to handle so much extra refined carbohydrates.

Fats help us to feel satisfied, so that we know when to stop eating. We will need to eat just a little fat with each meal, as this will help us to overcome carbohydrate cravings. The body seeks fat and will not stop eating until it gets what it needs. I am talking about the correct sort of fat, and I am certainly not suggesting you eat loads of it.

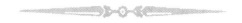

Chapter 23

Low Self-Esteem and Depression

"You don't have to cook fancy or complicated masterpieces -
just good food from fresh ingredients"
Julia Child

Our mood-enhancing brain chemicals are dependent on getting enough amino acids, found in protein foods and beans, plus whole grains. Due to the lack of good quality protein and, very importantly, certain nutrients that produce these mood-enhancing chemicals, the body turns to a quick-fix solution. It demands refined carbohydrates and sugars, in the absence of a good supply of amino acids and nutrients.

Serotonin, our Natural Prozac

The B Vitamins and zinc are important, as they help the brain to manufacture neuro-chemicals out of amino acids. A good supply of B3 is very important (found in whole foods), otherwise our body will make it out of tryptophan. You want to reserve your store of tryptophan for the production of serotonin, and not for making B3.

Eating foods that contain a good amount of tryptophan as well as the B Vitamins will ensure better levels of serotonin.

These foods are a good source of tryptophan:
- seeds - pumpkin, sunflower, sesame
- nuts - hazelnuts and almonds
- wild game
- chicken
- turkey
- bananas

· prawns
· yogurts.

By naturally enhancing our serotonin levels and by stabilizing our blood sugar levels, we will not be tempted to use 'quick-fix', empty calorie foods that are so addictive.

Casein and Gluten

Casein (the protein in cow's milk) and gluten (large amounts in wheat, smaller amounts in rye, and much smaller amounts in barley and oats), stimulate the production of exorphins, opiate chemicals very similar to endorphins. Over time we become addicted to these brain chemicals. Once hooked, going without could leave you feeling very uncomfortable.

Gluten ('glue') is very hard to digest. Gluten can actually inflame and even damage our digestive lining very easily. In its extreme, it can cause celiac disease (CD). I am not suggesting you are celiac, but for some people wheat (which contains the most gluten) is extremely addictive and can cause irritation or damage to the lining of our digestive tract. Once you cut down or remove wheat from your diet you may very well find other foods will be easier to digest, as the lining of your digestive tract improves and, of course, so does absorption. It's important that we not only digest our food well, but also absorb the nutrients we need.

Beware of the new low-carbohydrate trend and the 'low-carb' foods being touted as healthy. They have very large amounts of gluten added to them! Wheat is a grain, a source of carbohydrate, and the gluten is the protein part, which is very hard to digest. Think of chewing gum and you are close to imagining the texture of gluten! As I mentioned earlier in the book, most people eat wheat and hence large amounts of gluten each and every day. There is nothing to recommend it.

Wheat also contains phytic acid, which blocks the absorption of minerals like calcium and iron.

Most wheat products are made from refined white flour. Products that have had their nutrients removed are hard to digest, they irritate the digestive lining, hinder absorption of nutrients and, adding insult to injury, we eat it to excess.

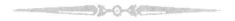

Chapter 24

Protein

"Man is what he eats"
Ludwig Feuerbach

Proteins help to keep our blood sugar levels even and in control. Before I go any further, I must stress that I am not an advocate of the high-protein diets that are so popular at the moment. However, the problem with people who are hooked on refined carbohydrates and sugar is that they generally don't eat enough protein-rich foods.

Protein foods trigger the release of glucagon, a hormone that provides a balance when excess carbohydrates trigger excess insulin. Glucagon stimulates fat burning instead of fat storage. It also discourages water retention, among other things. Protein stimulates glucagon activity and refined carbohydrates trigger the release of insulin, which results in fat storage and low blood sugar levels and cravings.

This doesn't mean you should start eating large amounts of protein - far from it, as you could end up with other health problems. Going from one extreme to another is never a good idea.

Protein Deficiency

One of the side effects of a low-protein diet and protein deficiency can be fluid retention. A 'low-fat' diet could easily mean low protein. Dieters often avoid nutritious foods like protein because of their fat content. Being hooked on refined carbohydrates leaves few 'points' or calories in a day's quota for protein and 'essential fatty acid' rich foods. I have seen many a 'life-long dieter' cringe in horror at the mere suggesting of adding raw nuts to their diets.

Protein-rich foods include:
- eggs (especially free-range or organic)
- fish
- meat
- nuts
- seeds
- avocados
- coconut
- normal yogurts
- goat milk cheese.

These protein-rich foods are important for replenishing your body's supply of all twenty-two amino acids. Our bodies can make some amino acids from other amino acids, but the essential amino acids need to be supplied through our food on a regular basis.

Amino acid deficiency symptoms include:
- cravings for sugar or alcohol
- moodiness
- depression
- lack of energy
- lack of drive
- lack of concentration
- inability to relax
- sensitivity and mood swings
- anxiety
- crying easily
- PMS
- disturbed sleep
- tense muscles
- fluid retention

Get Hydrated

Experiments have revealed that people often get confused between hunger and thirst, and will often eat when what the body really wants is something that will hydrate it. If you want to lose weight you will need to hydrate to switch off hunger.

These foods and drinks are dehydrating:

- tea
- coffee
- soft drinks
- alcohol
- salt
- sugar
- dry foods like bread, cakes, crisps, chocolate, biscuits, etc. (these are also the very foods and drinks that will mess up your blood sugar levels)
- a diet too high in protein.

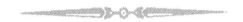

Chapter 25

The Program

"Getting my lifelong weight struggle under control has come from a process of treating myself as well as I treat others in every way"
Oprah Winfrey: O Magazine, August 2004

By now you should have started the food and symptom diary we mentioned earlier. Remember to weigh yourself only very occasionally - it's more important to measure yourself. People often remark how the scales haven't changed dramatically, yet their clothes are much looser. One kilo of muscle takes up less space than one kilo of fat. Also, you will need to be patient, as this kind of weight loss will take a bit longer than conventional weight-loss programs. This program is designed to sort out your health problems and solve cravings. It will give you a sense of well being with more energy, making you feel more positive, freeing you from yo-yo dieting with quick weight loss and, more importantly, the inevitable weight gain. It will enable you to be more in control. This program will take some getting used to, but once you have, it's easy and the benefits are huge. Habits of a lifetime are hard to change; it just takes a little time. Remember, there is no time limit to getting healthy and slimmer.

Avoiding the big three 'drug foods':
1. Wheat
2. Sugar
3. Dairy (with exceptions - natural yogurt, goat's and sheep's products)

After seeing this shortlist, you may look at your food diary and see plenty of entries for the three main foods mentioned above. You are probably contemplating, or maybe even panicking about what on earth you are going to eat in the future.

There are plenty of alternatives, most of which are very easy to find in many supermarkets and health shops.

1. Wheat

So, what products contain wheat?

- Breakfast cereals
- Baked products - breads, rolls, buns, pancakes, pizzas, croissants, crackers, pretzels, sweet biscuits, cakes, pies, doughnuts, etc.
- Pasta - noodles, macaroni, spaghetti, bulgar wheat, durum wheat, couscous.
- Soup - often thickened with flour or containing noodles.
- Others - batter, breadcrumbs (on fish or chicken), sausages, gravy, white sauces, soy sauce (use tamari, a wheat-free soy sauce).
- Hidden - MSG (monosodium glutamate), HVP (hydrolyzed vegetable protein), TVP (textured vegetable protein), mayonnaise, ketchup, distilled vinegar, caramel coloring, modified food starch, malt, sulfites, seitan (all gluten), baking powder (wheat-free can be found) and some tortillas.

So many foods are made from, or contain wheat. This is just one grain. As I am sure you are only too well aware, it isn't difficult to overdo it.

Yet, there are about a dozen grains to choose from! It makes you wonder, with so many grains in existence, why the world is full of wheat!

2. Sugar

Sugar, our other drug food, comes in many guises and is found in so many products these days. Many foods labeled 'low-fat' or 'no-fat' often contain sugar. Foods like baked beans or tomato ketchup contain plenty of sugar.

What do you need to look out for? First, anything with -ose on the end of the word:

- sucrose
- maltose
- dextrose

- glucose
- levulose
- galactose.

Then there are words ending in -ol:
- mannitol
- sorbitol
- xylitol.

Plus:
- corn syrup
- maltodextrins
- malt.

Even a good thing - taking more than a little occasionally will be bad for your blood sugar levels and addictive:
- maple syrup
- honey.

Changing from refined sugars to honey or pure maple syrup is only a very short-term strategy, as it's very important to re-educate your taste buds as soon as possible. You will be surprised how your taste buds will not be able to cope with so much sweetness in a relatively short time.

Gradually change your sweet snacks for fresh fruit or dried fruit. Remember you need to get into the habit of reading every label; it should become second nature. As time goes on the food you choose will have labels with very short ingredient lists or no label at all.

3. Dairy Products from Cows

These foods can be a problem for a lot of people. They can cause digestive problems, addictions and respiratory congestion of one type or another, such as sinus problems, runny nose, asthma and even earaches. You may have a problem with the milk protein casein, or the milk sugar lactose. Generally, but not always, the digestive problems of pain, wind, bloating, cramping, diarrhea or constipation are caused by lactose. Respiratory problems are usually caused by the protein casein.

What to look out for on labels:
· casein
· caseinates
· galactose
· whey protein
· whey
· lactose (sodium lactylate).

Other words that begin with lact-:
· lactalbumin
· lactoglobulin.

Still read the labels of foods that say 'non-dairy', 'milk free' or dairy free'. They may still contain plenty of casein and yet still meet the definition of 'dairy free'.

I recommend you use goat's milk products instead. Some of them taste wonderful. The protein alpha-casein found in large amounts in cow's milk is only found is tiny amounts in goat's milk. Like human milk, goat's milk contains beta-casein proteins, which are much easier for most of us to digest. The deli counters in many supermarkets sell several varieties of hard and soft goat and sheep cheeses from different parts of the world.

Yogurt is different, as it has been pre-digested by bacteria, making it much easier for us to digest. The beneficial bacteria in yogurt keep the body's digestive system working correctly. Use only natural 'live' yogurt. This habit will reintroduce the beneficial bacteria, so eating natural 'live' yogurt on a regular basis will help to keep certain yeasts, such as candida, from multiplying to harmful levels. Most people who are lactose intolerant will find they can eat natural yogurt, as long as it contains the active cultures only.

Twelve steps to Changing our Lifelong Habits

1. Skipping meals is a really bad habit. A lot of people regularly skip breakfast. Skipping breakfast will slow down your metabolism. It also encourages your blood sugar levels to drop. Skipping breakfast is playing with fire as you may well end up with cravings in the afternoon or overeating in the evening, or both! You need to manage your blood sugar levels carefully from now on. Some of the most popular breakfast foods raise blood sugar levels too high and

encourage insulin production and hence a drop later in the day, causing hunger, craving and guilt. The vicious circle continues. Look up the recipe section on breakfasts - you will find ideas for breakfast that will help maintain your 'blood sugar' levels.

2. No more calorie counting, no more malnourishment, no more self-starvation. We need to eat more food, but only food that is going to provide nutrients; only foods that keep our blood sugar levels stable. The brain and body will not switch off hunger if you are starving yourself of 'essentials'. Your body will encourage your appetite until it gets what it needs to keep your body functioning comfortably. You should consume twenty-five per cent of your daily intake at breakfast. It should contain protein of some description. Some people say they can't have breakfast because they don't have the time. Others have told me they don't have breakfast because they will be hungry soon after. This is due to their choice of food. From now on you need to make time, it's important to your health, your metabolism and your weight.

3. I need to remind you; this program isn't 'a diet' that you can 'come off'. It will become a way of life for life. I know it's hard to believe right now, but as time goes on, this program will become second nature. I now find it so easy not to eat anything made of white flour and other refined foods. In fact if I had to eat anything made of white flour I'd find it a punishment. You need to realize you are addicted to certain foods, that it's not just a matter of willpower.

4. The good news is, you'll be able to eat more (of the right foods), not less. Most dieters under-eat, and this is a problem.

5. Lunches and dinners also need to contain some protein, loads of vegetables or salad. If you feel the need, you can add a little of the right type of carbohydrate.

6. Snacking is important to keep your blood sugar levels stable, especially at first. Some of you will need to eat every two hours, but only foods that will maintain your blood sugar levels.

7. Pulses (beans and lentils) - use them in salads, soups, casseroles, curries, etc. They are a good source of protein, nutrients, fiber, and also carbohydrates. They are filling and low in fat naturally. Avoid soybeans, as they are extremely hard to digest, unless you eat them in the form of tofu or tempeh (fermented for easier digestion). Eat pulses with whole grains; this is especially important if you are a vegetarian. If you have this type of meal, it isn't necessary to have

any other type of protein food.

8. Raw, fresh fruit is a fantastic source of fiber, fluid, vitamins, minerals and the all-important enzymes. Fruit contains fruit sugar called fructose. For a few of us, fruit can cause tiredness and cravings, but this is very unusual. If you are one of these rare people, then eat your fruit with a good portion of nuts, seeds, cheese or yogurt.

9. Any health program would be incomplete without endless amounts of vegetables. You will easily acquire a taste for them, as you give up your 'drug foods'.

10. Don't eat a big meal late in the evening.

11. To turn off your cravings and hunger, you need to:

- eat some protein at each meal, like fish, chicken, eggs, yogurt, or beans with whole grains, etc.
- snack on nuts and seeds or fresh fruit
- get enough good fats daily - fish, olive oil, butter, avocados, nuts and seeds
- drink enough hydrating fluids during the day
- eat enough fiber; it's filling and will remove excess estrogen

12. Eat plenty of enzyme-rich foods every day - this is important.

As a dieter, you will be used to being told how much to eat ,or, more correctly, how little to eat. I am often asked how much one should eat. No one really knows the answer to that, as we are all different. The World Health Organization has declared that on anything less than 2,100 calories a day, you are starving yourself. The smaller, thinner Chinese eat twenty per cent more calories than us in the West!

What Does your Body Need?

Surveys show that most people consume inadequate amounts of almost every vitamin and mineral, EPA, enzymes, fiber, and plant chemicals studied.

Here is what you should be consuming:
- water
- minerals
- vitamins
- enzymes
- essential fatty acids
- amino acids (protein)
- the right carbohydrates
- plant chemicals

Billions are spent each year to tempt us to buy processed foods, with plenty of addictive ingredients like salt, sugar or refined carbohydrates. We are fed half-truths, as the advertisers prey on our emotions. These large industries have some very clever scientists working for them. They know exactly what their foods are doing to us. Addictions are good for the food industry's bottom line. Coca-Cola is advertised as the 'real thing'. What does that mean? One thing I am sure they know is just how addictive their drink is.

When you study your food diary, you will have probably noticed:
1. You are not eating enough fresh fruit and vegetables. Surveys reveal that less than ten per cent of us get the minimum of five portions of fruit and vegetables. Fruit and vegetables are health-promoting and disease-preventing. They are highly nutritious, naturally low-calorie foods full of enzymes and are extremely cleansing.
2. You eat too much sugar, in one form or another. This will completely mess up your blood sugar levels, as do 3 and 4.
3. You skip too many meals in favor of snacking on things like chocolate, cakes or crisps, all downed with plenty of caffeine.
4. You have been eating refined white flour over and over again, in various products.

Eating Out

Parties. Some people say their biggest problem is parties or weddings. Foods at these venues tend to be refined wheat and more refined wheat. The way to cope with this situation is to eat before you go out. It's then so easy to refuse such foods when you're not hungry and your blood sugar levels are stable.

Restaurants. Going to a restaurant is usually not a problem. It's easy to get fish or meat or poultry with vegetables or salads. This should be enough food as a) you should not eat so much in the evening, and b) you should have eaten enough food throughout the day, to have kept your blood sugar levels balanced, so by the time you get to the restaurant you should not be starving. In my experience a lot of dieters starve themselves all day before going out to dinner in the evening. This is a bad idea, as by the time you get to the restaurant your blood sugar levels are so low, you will either choose the wrong things or eat too much.

Buffets. They are usually fine, with a choice of hot and cold meats, fish, seafood, salads, vegetables, fruit, and sometimes goat's cheese.

Out and about. Have a supply of nuts and seeds in your car, or at the office: if you find yourself unable to get anything suitable these nuts will stop you going for chocolate or something just as unsuitable. At least these nuts and seeds will keep you going for the time being, ensuring your blood sugar levels remain stable.

Fast food places. These can be problem - you just have to make the most of it. Most of them do salads and all do meat like burgers or chicken or fish; you just need to discard the bread. Having chips (French fries) will not be fatal on the odd occasion.

Lunch at work. If you work, the type of food you take will be dependent on whether you have access to a fridge, cooker or microwave (only if there is no alternative). A thermos flask is good for soup.

If there is no fridge at work, put your tuna, goat's cheese, chicken, beans, grains and salad in a small, insulated container (sold to keep drinks cold). If you have to, due to time constraints, make the salad the day before.

Take hummus (chickpea) or lentil dip/spread with veggie sticks, like celery, peppers, carrots, etc. Also take fresh fruit and nuts.

Breakfast

Breakfast is so important to get the metabolism going, to stave off hunger and start your blood sugar on the right path. You will need to have some protein at each meal.

Try one of the following:

·   Smoothies are quick and easy. Use yogurt and fresh fruit, and blend in a blender. Add a little water if necessary and some protein powder (found in health shops).

·   Natural yogurt with nuts, seeds and fresh fruit.

·   Eggs scrambled with leftover vegetables or frozen vegetables.

·   Porridge made with water, with a little dried fruit to sweeten if needed. Then, once on your plate, add natural yogurt and linseeds.

·   Leftovers from the day before from lunch or dinner.

·   Goat's cheese with rice cakes or any special bread, i.e. whole grain rye, spelt or sprouted.

If you are not used to eating breakfast, then start off with a smoothie. If even this is a problem for you, then I think you may well be having caffeine first thing.

Caffeine disrupts your blood sugar levels and appetite. Have the smoothie first and give up caffeine as soon as possible. Remember, decaf has some caffeine.

Main Meals at Home

Eating lunch at home is far easier. You just have to make sure you make time for lunch and dinner.

We have already discussed:

·   fish
·   meat
·   poultry
·   eggs
·   seafood
·   tofu
·   beans and whole grains
·   all with loads of vegetables or a large salad
·   plus brown rice (or other whole grains) or maybe a jacket potato.

Bread

If you have a bread maker, spelt flour is a great substitute for wheat. Add protein powder and seeds like sunflower seeds or linseeds.

Always cook more - for instance, while baking salmon or pieces of chicken for dinner, cook an extra one for lunch. Making a veggie frittata bigger than you would normally, keeping some for the next day. In my experience if you have that piece of salmon or chicken ready to eat at lunch with an easy to prepare salad, it will be easy to avoid those foods you ate in the past. Being organized is more than half the battle.

As with any addiction, there can be withdrawal symptoms, but not always.

Side Effects

Some people can feel better straight away but others may suffer:
· headaches
· tiredness
· anxiety
· even stronger cravings
· irritability
· diarrhea, constipation or both
· restless sleep.

These symptoms can last two or three days normally, but for some people it can take as long as a week before you begin to feel good. Warn your family, friends and work colleagues.

Do not start this program the week before a period.

Continue to write your food and mood diary.

In a Nutshell

Weight loss should be slow if we want to maintain the loss. Our first priority is getting our health restored.

The key is to:
· nourish your body,
· stabilize your hormones
· take the stress off your organs
· manage your blood sugar levels
· hydrate.

It's important not to raise your blood sugar levels. We don't want to promote insulin production, as it will encourage us to eat the wrong foods, to overeat, enhance cravings and lay down body fat.

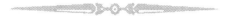

Part Four

In The Kitchen

Chapter 26

Recipes

"A watched pot never boils"
19th cent.

Our bodies are composed entirely from molecules derived from our food. In your lifetime you will eat 100 tons of food, which could either nourish you or leave you depleted. If your internal environment is too hostile due to poor food choices, you cannot adapt and disease can result. If you are correctly nourished, you will have a greater resistance to disease and are more likely to experience health and vitality.

The Basics

Egg Substitute
(if you have a problem with eggs)
12fl oz (300ml) water
6oz (170g) dried apricots or dates
Cook until soft, then puree.
2 tablespoons = 1 egg in cake recipes.
This recipe can be used in cakes for children.
It can be stored in the fridge for about three days.

Butter/Oil Spread

½lb or 225g butter

8fl oz or 225ml cold-pressed olive oil

Cut butter into cubes and cream by hand or in a blender. Mix in the oil gradually, a few drops at a time, until creamy and smooth.

The mixture of butter and oil can be kept in the fridge as long as you would normally keep butter. Kept cool, butter has about 1 or 2 months' shelf life.

Breakfast

Wheat-Free Muesli

Oat flakes, barley flakes, brown rice flakes, millet flakes, amaranth flakes, quinoa flakes, pumpkin seeds, linseeds, dried fruit and nuts.

Use in any combination you wish.

Combine all ingredients, mix well and store in an airtight container.

Take two heaped tablespoons or more per person, and place the muesli in a bowl. Add water to about half an inch or 1cm above the muesli. In the morning the muesli should be soft but not swimming in water; if this is the case, add less water the next time. Then add natural 'live' yogurt and/or fresh fruit to the soft, moist muesli.

It's very important to soak the grains before you eat your muesli. Soaking the grains overnight activates enzymes, making the grains much easier to digest. The grains will also expand in your bowl instead of your stomach.

Gluten-Free Muesli

Leave out oat and barley flakes from the wheat-free recipe above. This must also be pre-soaked.

Muesli Porridge

110g wheat-free muesli (without yogurt, fruit or nuts)

280ml water

Pre-soak the muesli in water overnight. In the morning add a little more water, if necessary.

Cook over a gentle heat for about 15 to 20 minutes, stirring most of the time. Once in your bowl, you can add yogurt, nuts and seeds.

Quick Porridge

85g oat flakes
Dried fruit, seeds (optional)
340ml water or water/rice milk mixture
Or follow the manufacturer's instructions.

Soak the oats in half the water overnight. In the morning, add the rest of the water and cook gently, stirring to prevent burning and lumps. Serve hot, and add seeds, fruit, etc. Makes one serving.

Gluten-Free Porridge

Brown rice flakes
Follow recipe for porridge above

Quinoa with Oats (Gluten-Free)

1 cup quinoa, soaked
1 cup rolled oats
Dried fruit, nuts, seeds (optional)
3 cups water

Place all ingredients in a pot, and cover. Bring to the boil, then reduce heat and simmer for 30 minutes. Check regularly to ensure it doesn't stick to the bottom of the pan. Turn off heat; let it stand for 5 minutes with closed lid. Add fruit, yogurt, nuts or seeds. Makes four servings.

Brown Rice Breakfast Dish (Gluten-Free)

340g cooked brown rice (left over from night before)
270ml of water or water/rice milk mixture
Optional ingredients:
Nuts, seeds, dried or fresh fruit
Natural yogurt

Put rice and water/milk in a pot and stir over a medium heat until it thickens and the rice is soft. Remove from the heat and then add optional ingredients. Makes two to three servings.

Whole Millet or Quinoa (Gluten-Free)

750ml water

200g whole millet or Quinoa

Put ingredients in a pot, bring to the boil, cover and simmer for 8 to 15 minutes, checking regularly.

Millet can be used like porridge or with a main meal instead of rice, couscous, stuffing, or potatoes. Makes two to three servings.

Original Swiss Muesli

3 tablespoons medium oats

½ tablespoon oat bran

Water

Any milk of your choice, or yogurt

Dried or fresh fruit, chopped if necessary

1 tablespoon chopped nuts

Soak the oats and bran overnight in the water. If necessary, in the morning, add a little milk or yogurt. Then add your dried or fresh fruit and nuts, if you want. Makes one serving.

Fruit Salad

Any fresh fruit, chopped up and placed into a bowl and add yogurt, nuts and/or seeds.

Eggs

Eggs can be eaten scrambled or boiled, or as an omelet with vegetables (can be left over from the night before) and a little goat's cheese.

Serve with rice cakes, oatcakes, or 100% whole grain sourdough rye bread, spelt bread or sprouted bread.

Dips and Spreads

Cut up pieces of fresh, raw vegetables - carrots, cauliflower, broccoli, courgettes, various peppers, cucumber, celery, fennel, chicory, etc. to dunk into the dips.

You can also use rice crackers, rice cakes, oat biscuits and tortillas (which are made from cornmeal).

Lentil Pâté

1-2 teaspoon of extra virgin oil

2 onions, finely chopped

225g cooked red lentils

1-2 tablespoons tahini (sesame seed butter)

2 tablespoons chopped parsley or any combination of herbs
you want

Heat the olive oil and very lightly sauté the onions, without browning. Combine all ingredients and stir until the texture is thick and smooth. Allow the mixture to cool a little and puree if necessary. Add some cold-pressed oil or a little water if the mixture is too dry. Makes 4 servings.

Avocado Pâté

225g soft goat's cheese or tofu

1 large avocado pear

Juice of half a lemon

Fresh coriander

Peel and stone the avocado and blend all ingredients in a blender. Alternatively, blend by hand with a fork. Chill until required. Makes 4 servings.

Guacamole (Mexican Avocado Dip)

2 ripe avocados

1 tomato, peeled and finely chopped

Juice of a lemon - half to a whole, depending on taste

Chili, fresh or dried, or a little Tabasco

Blend all ingredients by hand until smooth. Makes 4 servings.

Chickpea Spread (Hummus)

225g chickpeas
2-4 tablespoons tahini (sesame seed butter)
2 garlic cloves, crushed
Juice of 1 large lemon

Soak the chickpeas overnight in sufficient water to cover well. Drain.

Place in a saucepan with just enough water to cover. Add the garlic and bring to the boil. Cover and simmer for 30 minutes or more until they are soft. Allow to cool in the water.

Put oil, lemon juice and tahini into a liquidizer/blender. Add half the chickpeas and garlic with the cooking liquid, then blend until smooth. Keep adding chickpeas, along with some water if needed, until the texture becomes creamy.

Put into a serving dish and keep in the fridge for a few hours.

For an easy life, I make triple the amount and divide into small containers for the freezer. Makes 4 servings.

Aubergine (Eggplant) Pâté

2 aubergines
Juice of 1 lemon
1-2 tablespoons tahini
Any herb
2 teaspoons olive oil

Preheat the oven to 200°C, 400°F. Prick the aubergines with a fork.

Roast until slightly charred (about 45 minutes), then allow to cool. Scoop out the middle and mash well. Combine all the ingredients except the olive oil.

Transfer to a bowl and drizzle the oil on top. Makes 4 servings.

Vegetable and/or Bean Spread

1 cup cooked vegetables and/or beans
1 teaspoon miso (optional)
1 tablespoon tahini
Cooked chopped onion
1 tablespoon chopped parsley or other herbs
Spices of your choice
A little chopped coriander

Mash the vegetables/beans with a fork. Mix with the other ingredients. Serve as a dip, sandwich or in pancakes. Makes 2 servings.

Bread Recipes

Spelt or Rye Soda Bread (yeast-free)

8oz or 225g rye flour or spelt flour (or an equal mix of each)

1 level teaspoon bicarbonate of soda

¼ pint or 123ml water

1 tablespoon olive oil

This bread is very easy and quick to make.

Sieve flour and bicarbonate of soda together. Add the other ingredients and mix into dough.

Turn out onto a lightly floured surface and knead. Form into a round loaf and cut a large cross into the dough.

Place on a baking tray and bake at 230°C, 450°F for 15 minutes, then turn down to 200°C, 400°F and bake for a further 10 or 15 minutes.

Turn out and leave to cool on a wire rack.

Welsh Barley Bread

680g barley flour

Pinch of salt

1 packet of dried yeast (or fresh)

A little warm water

2 tablespoons molasses

450ml lukewarm water

1 tablespoon olive oil

Put yeast and molasses in a bowl with a little warm water and set aside to froth. Put the flour and salt into another bowl then add the frothed yeast liquid, the lukewarm water and the oil. Mix to make dough. Knead well on a floured surface.

Place in a warm place for about 2 hours, until it doubles its size.

Knead again and place in a large greased tin, cover and leave to rise (prove) again for an hour.

Then, make a deep cut along the loaf. Bake at 200°C, 400°F for approx 1 hour.

Potato and Rice Bread (Gluten-Free)

285g potato flour
225g brown rice flour or buckwheat flour
250ml hand-hot water
4 teaspoons dried yeast
1 teaspoon muscovado sugar
1 tablespoon olive oil

Put the sugar and dried yeast into the water and leave in a warm place to form a froth about 1 inch, 1.5cm deep.

Put the flour and the salt in a large bowl and then add the yeast liquid with the oil. Mix into a thick batter, adding more warm water if the mixture is too thick.

Oil two 1lb loaf tins, then flour freely to prevent loaves from sticking. Divide mixture into the two tins. Leave to rise in a warm place for 20 to 30 minutes.

Bake at 230°C, 450°F for 35 to 40 minutes. Turn out and leave to cool on a wire rack.

Chickpea Bread (Gluten-Free)

505g chickpea flour (gram flour)
500ml hand-hot water
4 teaspoon dried yeast
1 teaspoon muscovado sugar
50g butter

Put the sugar, dried yeast and hand-hot water into a jug and leave in a warm place until the froth is about an inch or 1.5cm high.

Mix the flour and salt together in a large bowl and rub the butter into the flour. Add the yeast fluid and mix to a thick batter, adding more warm water if necessary.

Grease two 1lb loaf tins and flour well with chickpea flour. Divide the mixture between the two tins. Leave in a warm place for 20 to 30 minutes.

Bake at 230°C, 450°F for 35 to 40 minutes. Turn out to cool on a wire rack.

Gluten-free breads should be eaten fresh or kept in the freezer and then toasted.

Millet Bread (Yeast-Free and Gluten-Free)

110g millet flour

1 medium-sized carrot, grated

1 tablespoon honey or molasses

2 tablespoons cold water

200ml boiling water

2 tablespoons olive oil

2 eggs

Pinch of salt

Combine the millet flour, grated carrot, molasses or honey, salt and oil. Mix well.

Stir in the boiling water.

Separate the eggs and beat the whites until stiff. Beat the yolks well, add two tablespoons of cold water and continue to beat.

Add this fluid to the flour mixture, and mix well. Then fold in the stiffly beaten egg whites.

Place this batter in an oiled oblong baking tin and bake at 180°C, 350°F for about 45 minutes. Turn out to cool on a wire rack.

Rice, Soya and Dried Fruit Bread
(Yeast-Free and Gluten-Free)

170g brown rice flour or millet four

55g soy flour

4 tablespoons soy milk or goat's, sheep's, or rice milk

2 eggs

4 tablespoons oil

4 tablespoons honey or molasses

2 teaspoons wheat-free baking powder

55g natural raisins or chopped apricots

30g chopped nuts or seeds

Mix milk, eggs, honey or molasses and oil.

Sieve all dry ingredients and gradually blend into the mixture.

Stir in the raisins and nuts. Pour into a well-oiled bread tin and leave to rest for 1 hour.

Bake at 180°C, 350°F for about 45 minutes, checking from time to time. Turn out and cool on a wire rack.

Corn Meal Bread (Yeast-Free)

225g corn maize meal

1 level teaspoon bicarbonate of soda

250ml goat's, sheep's, soy, or rice milk

3 tablespoons olive oil

1 egg

Brush an 8- or 9-inch, 20-cm tin with oil.

Blend all ingredients together well. Pour into tin.

Bake at 220°C, 425°F for 20 to 25 minutes.

Cut into squares while still in the tin and then transfer to a wire rack to cool.

Cakes, Biscuits/Cookies, etc.

Even though these are a healthier alternative, eat only occasionally as a treat. Really good for children, though.

Pastry (Gluten-Free)

225g buckwheat, brown rice or chickpea flour

½ teaspoon wheat-free baking powder

5 tablespoons olive oil

3 tablespoons cold water

Whisk oil and water together. Put all ingredients into a large mixing bowl and work together to form a soft dough. This pastry is quite difficult to handle, so put the dough into an oiled pie dish and work it with the hands to cover the entire surface. Bake at 200°C, 400°F until cooked. Makes enough for one open pie.

Filling

Berries of various kinds

Peaches with a little ginger

Pears and cloves

Apples and cinnamon

Apple Pie Filling

5 to 6 medium cooking or green apples, sliced
55g dried fruit any of your choice
1 tablespoon water
½ teaspoon cinnamon or mixed spice
1 tablespoon arrowroot or kuzu (optional)

Stew apples and dried fruit gently in a little water. When mixture is soft add cinnamon or mixed spice. Dissolve arrowroot in a tablespoon of cold water. Use with oatmeal crust to make a pie.

Oatmeal Crust

340g rolled oats
110g barley or other flour
2 tablespoons oil
280ml water
Pinch of salt

Combine the oats and the flour with salt, add the oil and mix well.
Add the water and mix it into a stiff dough.
Roll out, place in a greased pie tin and bake blind at 275°F, 190°C for 10 minutes, or use to cover a pie.

Baked Cheesecake (Gluten-Free)

450g goat's or sheep's curd cheese or tofu
1 egg white, beaten
110g muscovado sugar
Fresh lemon juice
30g sultanas or other chopped dried fruit
Pastry recipe (above)

Line the bottom of a 7-inch, 18cm square tin or slightly bigger round tin with the pastry.
Put all ingredients in a bowl and mix well. Turn into the pastry-lined tin.
Bake at 190°C, 375°F for 45 to 50 minutes. Cool for 30 minutes in the tin, then when set take out and place on a wire rack. Makes 6 to 8 servings.

Carob or Cocoa Cake

110g butter
2 tablespoons honey or molasses
35g muscovado sugar
2 eggs
28g carob or cocoa powder
100g barley flour or a mixture of flours
1 teaspoon wheat-free baking powder
55g pumpkin seeds and/or nuts
55g sultanas
Cold water

Preheat the oven to 350°F, 180°C.

Lightly grease an 8-inch (20cm) cake tin and dust with flour.

Cream the butter, molasses and sugar, then beat in the eggs.

Add the carob or cocoa powder, the flour and the baking powder.

Add nuts and sultanas with enough water to give a dropping consistency.

Transfer the mixture to the tin and bake in the center of the oven for 20 to 25 minutes. Allow to cool slightly before turning out onto a wire rack. Makes 6 to 8 servings.

Ginger Spice Cake

110g whole barley flour, spelt flour or rye flour
55g rice flour
55g corn flour
1 teaspoon baking powder
½ teaspoon or more of mixed spice
½ teaspoon or more of dried ginger
2 or more cardamom seeds, crushed (optional)
110ml olive oil
55g honey
1 tablespoon molasses
170g dried fruit
1 egg, beaten

Mix together all dry ingredients. Mix the oil, honey and molasses together, then stir into the flour.

Add the dried fruit and then the beaten egg. Mix to a fairly stiff consistency, add a little water if necessary.

Place the mixture in an oiled 9-inch, 21-cm cake tin. Bake at 180°C or 350°F for about 45 minutes to an hour. Check regularly. Makes 6 to 8 servings.

Boiled Fruit Cake

55g butter
55g olive oil
110g muscovado sugar or molasses
170g currants
170g sultanas
60g chopped apricots
55g candied peel
28g glacé cherries
225ml water
1 level teaspoon baking soda
1 level teaspoon mixed spice
2 beaten eggs
225g whole barley flour or spelt or mixture of flours

*Place all ingredients except the eggs and flour in a pan and boil for 1
minute. Allow to cool.*

Add eggs and flour and beat well. Bake at 375°F, 190°C for 1¼ hours.

This is really quick and easy to make. Makes 6 to 8 servings.

Flapjacks

140g butter
2 tablespoons honey
28g muscovado sugar
225g rolled oats

Lightly grease an 8-inch (20-cm) square, shallow cake tin.

Gently heat the butter, honey and sugar in a pot until melted.

Stir in the oats, remove from the heat and turn mixture into a tin.

Bake in the oven until golden at 350°F or 180°C.

These are good for children's lunch boxes, as well as being quick and
easy to make.

As a variation, you could reduce oats and add nuts or seeds and/or dried
fruit. Makes 8 servings.

Seed Biscuits (Gluten-Free)

170g freshly ground seeds or almonds
110g brown rice flour
1 tablespoon honey or molasses
2 tablespoons olive oil
1 apple, grated
2 tablespoons ice-cold water

Mix all ingredients together well. Knead the mixture, roll into balls and flatten on an oiled baking tray.

Bake for 30 minutes at 350°F, 180°C, then allow them to cool on a wire rack. Good for children's lunch boxes.

Apple and Dried Fruit Dessert (Gluten-Free)

110g dried fruit - apricots, peaches, sultanas, prunes, etc
455g cooking or dessert apples
Mixed spice or cinnamon, cloves and juniper berries
100ml plain yogurt

Soak the dried fruit overnight.

Stew the apples and the soaked dried fruit together with the spices until tender. Eat with natural yogurt. Makes 4 servings.

Creamy Rice Pudding (Gluten-Free)

340g cooked short-grain brown rice
840ml rice, soy or goat's milk
½ teaspoon honey or molasses (optional)
½ teaspoon of spice
110g flaked almonds
110g sultanas or raisins or apricots

Combine all the ingredients and bake in the oven at 350°F, 180°C for 1 hour. Serve hot or cold. Makes 4 servings.

Chocolate or Carob Biscuits

85g butter

55g molasses or muscovado sugar

1 egg, beaten

255g brown rice flour or a mixture of flours

30g pure cocoa powder or carob powder

Cream together the butter and sugar until light and fluffy.

Beat in the egg gradually. Stir in flour and cocoa or carob powder.

Knead on a lightly floured surface. Roll out thinly and cut into circles with a 2-inch, 3-cm biscuit cutter.

Place on a greased baking tray, leaving room to spread, and bake at 160°C, 325°F for about 20minutes.

Cool slightly before transferring to a wire rack to cool completely.

Sugar-Free Cake

225g brown rice, or millet flour, or a mixture of flours

1 level teaspoon bicarbonate of soda

1 teaspoon ground ginger

250ml goat's, sheep's or soymilk

4 tablespoons olive oil or coconut oil

85g grated coconut

2 eggs, beaten

Mashed banana

Grated apple

Apricots soaked overnight, cooked and pureed

Brush an 8- or 9-inch, 20-cm square or oblong cake tin with oil.

Blend or whisk all ingredients well. Pour into the tin and bake at 220°C, 425°F for 20 to 25 minutes. Cut into squares whilst still in the tin and then transfer to a rack to cool. Makes 6 to 8 servings.

Pineapple Pudding

1 small ripe pineapple
Strawberries or raspberries
225g goats' or sheep's curd cheese

Wash pineapple and other fruit; dry on kitchen paper.

Cut pineapple into quarters lengthways, scoop out flesh and chop.

Place cheese in a bowl and stir in pineapple. Pile into pineapple 'shells' and decorate each with the other fruit.

Put on a serving dish; keep cool until ready to serve. Makes 4 servings.

Carob or Cocoa Dessert

375-500ml goat's, sheep's, soy, oat or rice milk
2 level teaspoons agar
2 tablespoons molasses
1 tablespoon carob or cocoa powder
A few drops of natural vanilla

Dissolve agar in a little hot water. When dissolved add enough milk to make 500ml.

Pour into a liquidizer with the other ingredients and blend until smooth.

Pour into a dish and leave to set. Makes 4 servings.

Buckwheat Crêpes (Gluten-Free) 1

170g buckwheat flour
¼ teaspoon cinnamon or mixed spice
1 egg, well beaten
570g water

Combine the dry ingredients. Add the egg and water to form a thin smooth batter.

Heat a heavy pan, brush lightly with oil. Put enough batter into the pan to cover the surface thinly.

Brown both sides. Serve with steamed vegetables, cooked onions, herbs, etc or fresh fruit and yogurt. Serves 4.

Buckwheat Crêpes (Gluten-Free) 2

50g buckwheat flour

50g rice flour

Pinch of salt

1 egg

300ml goat's sheep's, soya, rice or oat milk

Place the buckwheat, rice flour and salt in a bowl and make a well in the center of the flour.

Break in the egg and add a little of the milk, beating well with a wooden spoon. Gradually beat in the remaining milk, drawing the flour in from the sides to make a smooth batter.

Heat a little oil in a 7-inch, 18-cm non-stick frying pan.

Pour in enough batter to coat the base of the pan thinly.

Cook until golden brown, then turn and cook on the other side.

Serve with savory things or fruit. Serves 4.

Carob or Cocoa Banana Cream Boats

250g tofu or soft goat's cheese

8 bananas, peeled

Fresh fruit like strawberries, raspberries or blueberries

2 teaspoons cocoa powder or carob powder

2 handfuls pumpkin seeds or chopped nuts

A few tablespoons rice, oat, goat's or sheep's milk

Put the cheese and two bananas (or if using tofu, roughly chop up the tofu and two bananas), then whiz in a blender with the cocoa or carob powder, pumpkin seeds or nuts and some milk until the mixture is creamy.

Cut the remaining six bananas lengthways into halves and place on a plate in pairs.

Cover one half with the chocolate cream and press the two halves together to make a boat shape.

Decorate with fruit and nuts or seeds, etc.

This cream can be used with a variety of dishes.

Yogurt Ice-Cream (Gluten-Free)

450g ripe fresh fruit

600ml natural yogurt

A little honey or maple syrup or pureed dried fruit (soaked in water)

Place fruit in a blender or food processor and blend until smooth. Transfer to a bowl, add the yogurt and mix well.

Add some sweetness to taste, only if necessary. Pour into a shallow plastic container.

Cover and place in the freezer for about 1½ to 2 hours until mushy.

Now beat until smooth. Return to freezer.

To serve, put into the fridge for 30 minutes beforehand to allow it to soften a little.

Though this ice-cream is more healthful than bought ice-creams, a lot, but not all of the beneficial bacteria in the yogurt, are destroyed in the freezing process.

Buy an ice-cream maker, if you have children, to make life easier. That way, you will know what your children are eating, as you will have put natural healthy ingredients into their ice-cream.

Pumpkin Pie (Gluten-Free)

1 medium pumpkin or squash

1 tablespoon honey

½ a bar of firm tofu or goat's or sheep's cream cheese

1 cup of flour, like brown rice flour

½ teaspoon each of cinnamon, ginger and cloves

¼ teaspoon nutmeg

¼ teaspoon sea salt

Enough pastry to line two dishes

Peel and cut the pumpkin into small pieces and put into a pan. Add honey.

Cover and cook until tender. Add a little water if needed.

Add puréed tofu during the last 10 minutes of cooking, or add the cream cheese at the end.

Mix all ingredients together really well.

Pour into the pie crusts and bake for 1 hour at 300°F.

This recipe makes two pies.

Tofu Pie

1 cake of firm tofu
2 tablespoons tahini
¼ cup honey and/or ¼ cup molasses
Juice of a lemon
fresh grated ginger
¼ teaspoon sea salt (optional)
1½ teaspoon vanilla
Pastry, baked blind

Preheat oven to 350°F or 180°C.
Puree all ingredients together. Pour into the pie crust.
Bake 30 to 35 minutes, until the top is lightly golden.
Cool and top with fruit.
You could use crystallized ginger, in which case, use less honey.
Makes about 6 servings.

Vegetables

You will have, no doubt, a lot of recipe books with interesting ways of cooking vegetables, but here are a few of my favorites.

Spiced Cabbage

1 medium cabbage, chopped
½ teaspoon caraway seeds
1 teaspoon each of ground coriander, cumin and fresh grated
    ginger
¼ teaspoon turmeric
Some coconut milk

Place all the ingredients into a saucepan and simmer on a low heat for
*   30 minutes until the cabbage is tender. Makes 2 servings.*

Brussels Sprouts with Pine Nuts

500g Brussels sprouts

½ cup pine nuts or pumpkin seeds

1 teaspoon thyme or any herb of your choice

1 teaspoon freshly grated ginger

½ small cup of miso, water or a little wine

Steam the sprouts. Put the miso, thyme and ginger in a pan and boil for a short while.

Arrange the Brussels sprouts on a dish and pour over the mixture.

Then, sprinkle over nuts or seeds. Makes 2 servings.

Veggie Curry

1 onion, chopped

A little olive oil

1 bay leaf, broken

1 green or red chili, chopped

1 garlic clove, minced

1 inch of ginger, grated

½ teaspoon turmeric

Sea salt and pepper

500mg of carrots cubed

½ cauliflower or broccoli, broken into florets

1 cup green beans

1 teaspoon each of coriander and cumin seeds

1 cup coconut milk

Gently sauté the onions and garlic. Add all the remaining ingredients and gently cook on a low heat until the vegetables are tender. Makes 4 servings.

Spiced Red Cabbage

2 tablespoons olive oil
1 teaspoon ground coriander
500g red cabbage sliced thinly
large onion
2 large cooking apples, peeled and chopped
5 cloves
2 bay leaves
1 tablespoon muscovado sugar
2 tablespoons apple cider vinegar
110g walnuts
A little sea salt and black pepper

Put all the ingredients (except the walnuts) into a pot and cook on a low heat until soft, stirring occasionally.

Five minutes before the end of cooking, add the walnuts. Makes 2 servings.

Herby Lentil Rice

175g basmati rice
175g red lentils
35g butter
Large onion, sliced
2 garlic cloves, crushed
250g carrots, chopped
2 parsnips or any root vegetable, chopped
1 teaspoon ground cumin
2 bay leaves
2 cinnamon sticks
6 cloves
6 cardamom pods, bruised
600ml miso or water
1 ripe avocado, diced

Soak rice and lentils in cold water for 3 or 4 hours. Heat the butter and sauté the onions gently, until soft. Drain the rice and lentils. Put all the ingredients (except avocado) into a pot, bring to boil, cover and simmer until cooked. Add the avocado and serve immediately. Makes 4 servings.

Gluten-free Tabouleh

One cup quinoa, millet or amaranth

2 cups of water

Small handful of peas

½ cucumber, chopped

6 olives, chopped

A few chives, minced

Plenty of parsley or coriander, minced or chopped very fine

Juice of half a lemon

A little salt

Combine quinoa, water and salt in the pot. Cover and bring to the boil, then simmer for about 10 minutes.

Meanwhile, steam the peas.

Place all the ingredients in a bowl and mix together.

Makes 3 to 4 servings.

Baked Quinoa or Millet Loaf

3 cups cooked quinoa or millet

1 cup flour of your choice

½ cup water

1 tablespoon miso or a few spices of your choice

1 tablespoon lecithin granules or 1 to 2 eggs

1 teaspoon each of basil, parsley and thyme

1 onion, chopped

2 cups carrots or mixed vegetables, sliced

2 cups broccoli, chopped

1 tablespoon seeds of your choice

Steam the vegetables. Combine quinoa or millet and flour in a bowl.

Dissolve miso and lecithin in warm water (alternatively, dissolve the miso in a little tepid water, beat in the egg) and mix with the flour, quinoa or millet and herbs.

Mix in the vegetables and seeds, place in a baking dish.

Bake 30 to 40 minutes at 350°F or 180°C.

Makes 4 servings.

Spicy Rice

1 onion
A little butter or olive oil
340g long-grain brown rice
1 tablespoon miso dissolved in 750ml water
Turmeric to taste
2 teaspoons ground coriander
1 teaspoon ground cumin
1 teaspoon ground ginger
55g sultanas
55g raisins
1 bay leaf
85-110g almonds or other nuts (cashews are good for this
    recipe)
4 boiled eggs

*Peel, slice and finely chop the onion, then sauté gently in a little of the
    butter or olive oil until tender, not brown.*

*Stir rice into pan and cook for a minute. Gradually add miso water,
    sultanas, raisins, bay leaf and spices.*

*Cover pan and simmer for 30 to 35 minutes, stirring occasionally, until
    rice is tender.*

Stir in the nuts and remaining butter or oil and turn out onto a dish.

Shell the boiled eggs, cut in half length-wise and arrange on the rice.

Makes 4 servings.

Filling Food Recipes

Basic Polenta

1 cup polenta (coarsely ground yellow cornmeal)
3 cups water
A little salt

*Boil the water and gradually pour in the polenta. Stir while pouring.
    Bring to the boil.*

Add salt and cover. Simmer for 30 minutes. Stir very regularly.

*Pour into a dish and spread out to about 1/3 in. thick. You could use the
    cooked polenta as a pizza base, for your favorite pizza topping.*

*To serve, top with steamed or roasted vegetables, olive oil and a little
    goat's cheese and place in the oven until the cheese has melted.
    Makes 4 servings.*

Pizza Base

Polenta makes a good, gluten-free pizza base. See the
previous recipe.

Boiled Brown Rice

1 cup brown rice
1½-2 cups cold water
A little salt

Place rice, water and salt in a heavy pot with a tight lid. Bring to boil.
*Turn down heat and simmer for 25 to 45minutes, depending on the type
of rice. Check regularly.*
*To make life easier, cook double or treble or more and freeze some. Rice
is gluten-free. Makes 2 servings.*

Boiled Brown Rice and Lentils

1 cup brown rice and lentils (not the orange ones)
1½-2 cups cold water
A little salt

Follow cooking instructions for boiled brown rice, above.
Makes 2 servings.

Fried Rice

4 cups cooked rice
1 teaspoon olive oil
½ cup carrots, diced, or other vegetables
1 onion, chopped
1½ -2 cups boiling water

*Sauté the onion in the olive oil until soft but not brown, then add carrots
or vegetables for 3 minutes.*
*Add the rice with a tiny amount of water. Cook on a low heat for 15
minutes, adding the water a little at a time, until it has all been
absorbed and the rice is cooked. Don't brown. Makes 4 servings.*

Baked Rice

1 cup brown rice
2-3 cups boiling water
A little sea salt
½ teaspoon olive oil

Preheat oven to 350°F or 180°C. Place all ingredients in a baking dish. Cover and bake for 40-45 minutes or until the water is absorbed. Makes 2 servings.

Rice and Beans

2 cups brown rice
½ cup beans, soaked overnight and partly cooked
2 carrots, in chunks, or other chopped vegetables
1 teaspoon caraway, cumin, fennel, or dill seeds
Sea salt
4 cups boiling water

Place all the ingredients in a saucepan and cover. Simmer gently for 30 to 45 minutes until the rice is tender. Makes 4 servings.

Wild Rice

1 cup wild rice
4 cups water
Little sea salt

Place all the ingredients together in a pot, cover and bring to the boil.
Turn heat down to low and simmer for 25 to 45 minutes.
The rice is ready when the black grains have split open.
Drain off the liquid and save for soups. Makes 2 servings.

Multi-colored Rice

1 cup long-grain brown rice
½ cup wild rice
½ cup red rice
½ cup nuts or seeds
6 cups water
½ cup vegetables of your choice
1 onion, diced
1 tofu block, diced
2 teaspoons mixed dried herbs
A little salt and pepper

Preheat oven to 350°F or 180°C. Place water and rice in a casserole dish. Put the other ingredients, except the nuts, on top. Don't stir.

Cover and bake until all the water has been absorbed, about 1 to 1½ hours.

Now add the nuts.

Makes at least 4 servings.

Note: *Never re-boil rice, as it becomes toxic.*

Bits and Pieces

Lemon Sauce

¼ to ½ jar of tahini
½ cup water or miso
1 garlic clove, crushed
½ cup lemon juice
1 scallion or a few spring onions, minced
½ cup fresh parsley or coriander, minced
½ teaspoon cumin
1/2 teaspoon coriander powder

Combine all ingredients. Mix well in a blender. Makes 4 servings.

Mexican Salsa

2 medium tomatoes, diced
1 to 3 green chilies, minced
6 sprigs coriander leaves, chopped fine
Sea salt to taste
1 small onion, finely diced

Mix together and allow to stand for a minimum of 30 minutes before serving.

Serve with meat, vegetables or as a dip. Makes 4 servings.

Veggie Pasta Sauce

1 onion, minced finely
1 cup carrots, minced finely
1 garlic clove, minced finely
Celery, minced finely
Olive oil
4 parsnips, a yam or some pumpkin, cooked and pureed
2 tablespoons rice flour
Sea salt and pepper
Plenty of fresh chopped herbs
3 cups water

Gently sauté the onions and garlic, but don't brown.

Add 1 cup of water plus the carrots and celery, and simmer covered for 20 minutes on a low heat.

Now add the pureed vegetable and heat through.

Dilute the rice flour in 2 cups of water, add to the pot and simmer for another 10 minutes.

Add a lot of fresh herbs and simmer for another 5 minutes.

Serve over pasta or polenta or steamed vegetables. Makes 3 to 4 servings.

Home-Made Pesto Sauce

2 or 3 cups fresh basil leaves

½ cup pine nuts

2 garlic cloves

½ cup olive oil

4 tablespoons grated Parmesan cheese

Blend the basil and pine nuts in a food processor.

Add the oil a little at a time, then the cheese, until well blended and smooth.

Pour over pasta or steamed vegetables.

Stuffings

Most stuffing recipes call for breadcrumbs, but they are equally as good made with rice, millet, buckwheat, etc. Don't overcook the grain, as it will make the stuffing too sticky.

Quinoa, Amaranth or Millet with Nut Stuffing

2 tablespoons olive oil

2 onions, chopped finely

2 garlic cloves, crushed

1 celery stick, chopped

Cooked quinoa, amaranth or millet

1 to 2 teaspoons dried herbs

75g nuts

A handful of fresh parsley, chopped

Juice of half a lemon

Gently sauté the garlic, onions and celery until just soft.

Add dried herbs, quinoa, amaranth or millet and heat through.

At the last moment add the nuts, parsley and lemon juice, and season to taste. Makes 4 to 6 servings.

Rice Spice Stuffing

1 onion, diced
4 cups cooked brown rice
A little olive oil
1 teaspoon ground turmeric
2 teaspoons ground cumin
3 teaspoons ground coriander
2 teaspoons ground ginger
½ cup raisins
1 tablespoon of dried or fresh mint
Salt and pepper

Sauté the onion and continue to cook until soft, then add the spices, herbs (not the mint) and raisins.

Continue to cook for a few minutes.

Remove from the heat and add the mint. Stir this mixture into the brown rice.

This stuffing works well with chicken or shoulder of lamb.

Makes 4 to 6 servings.

Fish, Meat and Poultry

You will have plenty of cookbooks with recipes for chicken, turkey, venison, lamb, duck and fish, so I don't feel that it's really necessary to list any fish or meat recipes here. Just be sure to serve with plenty of vegetables - steamed, stir-fried or salads.

You won't need to go out and buy a load of new cookbooks, as it's very easy to convert your favorite recipes. It only takes a little practice and thought. However, I would recommend getting an Indian cookbook if you don't have one already, as they use plenty of herbs, spices, beans, lentils, meats, natural yogurt and different flours like gram flour (chickpea).

Soups

Soups are easy and convenient. Cook in a very large pot and freeze some for the days you are too busy to cook, or take some to work the next day. The possible combinations of vegetables, beans, grains, lentils, herb and spices are endless. All recipes serve 4 as a starter, and 2 as a main course.

Coconut and Vegetable Soup

1 onion, chopped
2 carrots, diced
1 small cauliflower, chopped
2 apples or pears, peeled, cored and diced
1 teaspoon each of cumin, coriander, turmeric and ginger
¼ teaspoon or more of chili powder
1 liter of miso or water
some cooked rice
2 tablespoons of grated coconut
3 tablespoons of chopped coriander leaves
Salt and pepper
Can of beans or a similar quantity of pre-cooked beans
Can or carton of coconut milk
Salt and pepper

Put onions and carrots into a tiny amount of water and cook until the onions are soft.

Add cauliflower, spices, apples and miso or water, bring to the boil and simmer until cooked.

Add the beans, rice coconut and the coconut milk; cook until the coconut has blended and the beans are heated through.

At the last minute, stir in the chopped coriander leaves.

Filling Soup

2 medium onions, chopped
350g cabbage, shredded finely
50g lentils
A good handful of cooked rice
1 liter miso or water
Rosemary and thyme to taste, or your favorite herbs
50g parmesan or hard goat's cheese
A little salt and pepper

Put onions and cabbage into a tiny amount of water and cook until onions are soft.

Add all ingredients, except the rice and cheese. Simmer until lentils are cooked.

Then, add the cooked rice, making sure it's cooked through, and finally add the cheese.

Bean Soup

250g beans of your choice, soaked overnight, drained and
    rinsed
2 onions, chopped
1 clove garlic, chopped
1 bay leaf
1 stick celery
Fresh mint, parsley, basil or any combination of fresh or dried
    herbs
2 carrots, chopped
1 liter miso or water
a little salt and pepper

Put all the ingredients into a pot, bring to the boil and simmer for 1½-2
hours until the beans are tender. Remove the bay leaf and puree the
soup.

Oriental Soup

25g dried Chinese mushrooms or 50g of any fresh mushrooms
25g spring onions, finely chopped
25g bamboo shoots (tinned) cut into matchsticks
25g Chinese cabbage (white cabbage will do) shredded finely
50g frozen peas
25g tofu, cut into matchsticks
1 to 2 (or more) red chilies, seeds and sliced
900ml miso or water
1 or 2 tablespoons tamari, if you are using water
3 tablespoons apple cider vinegar
2 teaspoons arrowroot
1 to 2 eggs, beaten
Salt and pepper

If using dried mushrooms, soak in some boiled water. Then drain, throw
away stalks and chop the caps thinly.
Place all the vegetables, water, vinegar and tamari into a pan and
simmer for 5 minutes.
Blend the arrowroot in a little water and add to the pan.
Stirring, bring to the boil, then reduce heat and simmer.
At the end, stirring really well, add the beaten eggs and serve
immediately.

Salads

Anything can be used to make a salad, not just tomatoes with some limp lettuce and a couple of slices of cucumber. Not an appetizing thought.

These are some of the things you can use - raw carrots, various radishes, chicory, rocket leaves, coriander leaves, cabbage, celery, various lettuces (pale green, red, round, long, dark green, curly or flat, small or large leaf, etc), fresh fennel bulb, asparagus, red or yellow peppers, chives, spring onions, cucumber, courgettes, cauliflower, celeriac, fresh beetroot, avocado, various sprouts, apple, pear, grapes, mango, pineapple, nuts, seeds, etc. You can also add fresh herbs and spices like ginger or chili, fresh basil or fresh coriander.

The combinations are endless. All recipes make 3 to 4 servings.

Oriental Salad

350g bean sprouts, or any other sprouts
125g grated coconut
1 grated Chinese radish or finely sliced Chinese cabbage
For the dressing:
Juice of 1 lemon
4 tablespoons cold-pressed sesame or olive oil
50g fresh ginger, grated
2 tablespoons sesame seeds
Sea salt
Place bean sprouts, coconut and radish/cabbage in a bowl. Put all the ingredients for the dressing together and mix well.
Pour over the salad and toss.

Ginger and Broccoli Salad

750g broccoli, steamed for 5 to 7 minutes
50g sesame or pumpkin seeds
For the dressing:
1 tablespoon honey
2 tablespoons olive oil
1 tablespoon tamari or soy sauce
1 to 2 teaspoons freshly grated ginger
1 garlic clove, crushed
Mix all the dressing ingredients together. Then pour over the broccoli and seeds while warm, and allow to cool.

Middle Eastern Salad

125g brown or green lentils, or whole buckwheat
500g green, white or Chinese cabbage, finely sliced
2 carrots, coarsely grated
1 tablespoon extra virgin oil
15g butter
250g onions, finely sliced
For the dressing:
1 tablespoon each of fresh lemon juice and oil
6 tablespoons natural yogurt
fresh mint, chopped
Sea salt and pepper

Cook lentils or buckwheat in 300ml of water until just tender and drain.
Sauté the onions in the oil and butter. Then mix the dressing and add all
the ingredients together.

Rocket and Pear Salad

Rocket leaves
Chicory leaves
2 ripe pears, thinly sliced
For the dressing:
Orange and lemon juice
A little honey
1 teaspoon dried tarragon or your favorite herbs
6 tablespoons natural yogurt or some olive oil

Mix the dressing and pour over the salad ingredients.

Courgette Salad

500g small courgettes, sliced
6 celery sticks, sliced
2 spring onions, sliced
125g green grapes, halved
For the dressing:
3 tablespoons apple cider vinegar or fresh lemon juice
2 tablespoons olive oil
Some grape juice

Make up the dressing and pour over the salad ingredients.

Fruity Tabouleh

250g millet or quinoa, cooked
6 tablespoons olive oil
Juice of 1 lemon
2 tablespoons chopped coriander
Lettuce
1 garlic clove, crushed
250g small courgettes, finely chopped
Grated carrots
Chopped fresh fruit

Simply toss all the ingredients together.

Green Salad

125g mixed green salad leaves
Sprouted alfalfa or cress or other sprouts
50g celery, sliced
50g spring onions, sliced
125g cucumber, sliced
2 crisp green eating apples, diced
1 ripe avocado, diced
6 tablespoons chopped herbs
4 to 6 tablespoons of salad dressing (see recipe below)
Chopped chives

Mix all the ingredients together in a large bowl.

Red Salad

250g red cabbage
1 can red kidney beans
125g radishes, sliced
strawberries or raspberries
1 red onion, sliced very thinly
200g beetroot, cut into thin strips
For the dressing:
2 tablespoons apple cider vinegar
A little muscovado sugar
2 tablespoons olive oil

Cover the cabbage with boiled water and leave for 5 minutes, then drain.
Mix the dressing ingredients together and pour over the salad.
Leave to stand for a while before serving.

Celeriac, Walnut and Apple Salad

1 celeriac (or celery, if celeriac is not available)
4 tablespoons lemon juice
Homemade mayonnaise (see recipe below)
3 eating apples, peeled, cored and diced just before serving
50g walnuts

Grate the celeriac coarsely and mix with mayonnaise and lemon juice straight away.
Add apples and walnuts just before serving.

Curried Pineapple and Avocado Salad

1 tablespoon olive oil
1 onion, chopped
2 teaspoons curry powder
1 small cucumber, chopped small
150ml water
2 tablespoons homemade mayonnaise (see recipe below)
4 tablespoons natural yogurt
1 pineapple, chopped (retaining the shells for serving)
1 large avocado, diced
4 sticks celery, thinly sliced

Sauté the onions in the olive oil with the curry powder, add the water and rapidly boil for 10 to 15 minutes, until it thickens.
Leave to cool, then stir in the mayonnaise and yogurt.
Add all the ingredients together, then pile on top of the pineapple shells.

Mayonnaise

2 egg yolks
1 teaspoon horseradish
300mg olive oil
Vinegar or lemon
Sea salt and pepper

Place egg yolks and horseradish in an electric blender, and work until smooth. With the machine running, pour the oil in very, very slowly, until the mixture is thick and creamy. Add the vinegar or lemon a drop at a time and blend for a few seconds. Add salt and pepper to taste.

Salad Dressing

Lemon juice or apple cider vinegar
Extra virgin olive oil
Fresh or dried herbs
Garlic or fresh ginger

If you are going to use vinegar instead of lemon juice, then only use apple cider vinegar.

The proportions of vinegar/lemon juice to oil will depend on your own taste.

Put all ingredients into a jar with a tight-fitting lid and shake well.

Keeps in the fridge for a couple of days.

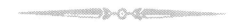

Chapter Twenty-Seven

Herbs and Spices

"The art of dining well is no slight art,
the pleasure not a slight pleasure"
Michel de Montaigne (1533 - 1592)

Culinary herbs and spices are every bit as therapeutic as the so-called 'medicinal' herbs and spices. This section will show you how easy it is to make your own medications for simple ailments, very cheaply. I am hoping this will open up a whole new way of thinking, and encourage you go on to find out more.

This is a simple introduction to the healing properties of the familiar herbs and spices you have been using in your cooking. It will give you an insight into how you can lead a healthier life, enhance your immune system, improve digestion and treat your own simple ailments without the use of over-the-counter pharmaceutical drugs.

The advice given in this book isn't meant to replace a practitioner's advice, especially in times of more serious complaints, such as allergies. If in doubt, always seek out the advice of a qualified herbalist, naturopath or your doctor. Never take herbs in therapeutic doses if you are pregnant, without seeking professional advice first. The small amounts of herbs and spices used in every-day cooking don't qualify as a 'therapeutic' dose. They are, nevertheless, enhancing your health.

Herbs have been categorized and divided into culinary or medicinal. This is not to say that the herbs and spices found in your kitchen cupboard don't have medicinal properties; they do. In some cultures they are one and the same. Looking after your health should be a way of life, it's far too important to leave to chance.

These herbs and spices can help to vastly improve our digestion and absorption. Some of them are also very nutritious, and will aid in the cleansing and detoxifying process. They are a very pleasant, convenient and cheap way of maintaining health.

Get into the habit of adding herbs and spices to whatever you are cooking.

If you are pregnant, only take therapeutic doses on the advice of a herbalist, naturopath or your doctor; don't self-prescribe. However, the little you use in cooking is not normally a problem, unless you are allergic to any of the ingredients.

AGE/STATUS	THERAPEUTIC DOSE
Average adult of about 10st 7lbs (147lbs)	As prescribed under each individual herb or spice
Up to the age of 5	¼ of the adult dose
From 6 up to the age 11	½ of the adult dose
From the age 11 to 17	¾ of the adult dose
For the elderly	Start off with ½ the adult dose and gradually increase
Pregnant	None unless advised. Amount in normal cooking is fine.
Regardless of age, start off any herbal program gradually!	

How to Take Herbs and Spices

Infusion
This is the simplest way of taking herbs therapeutically.

Equipment - A cup with a lid or a small teapot.

Measure -1 to 2 teaspoons of dried herb to 1 cup of boiled water.

Method - Pour boiling water over the herb, cover and let it steep for ten to twenty minutes.

Strain and drink one cup three times a day, unless it says otherwise under each individual herb.

Tip - To make life easier, you can make three cups in a teapot at one time. Drink one immediately and keep the other two in the fridge until needed.

Parts used - Leaves, flowers and seeds (if crushed a little before steeping).

Decoction

This method is used for the harder parts of the plant.

Equipment - Small saucepan (not aluminum).

Measure - 30gm (1oz) of dried herb.

Method - Place herbs and 750ml water into saucepan, bring to the boil and gently simmer for one hour. The liquid will have evaporated to approx 500ml. Strain and divide into three doses.

Tip - To make life easier make two days' worth if you want, but make sure you keep the rest in the refrigerator until needed.

Parts used - Roots, barks, twigs, berries and seeds.

Herbal Vinegar

Use a good quality apple cider vinegar, as it has healing properties the other types of vinegar don't have.

Equipment - A large glass jar with lid and smaller glass storage jars.

Measure - enough apple cider vinegar to cover the herb completely.

Method - Place dried herbs in a large jar and cover them completely with the vinegar. Shake every day for fourteen days, then strain and store in a glass container in a cool dark place.

Tip - Place the jar somewhere prominent, to remind you to shake it daily.

Parts used - Any part can be used.

Capsules

Good for herbs or spices that are too strong tasting to take in therapeutic doses, like cayenne.

Equipment - A shallow bowl and empty capsules. Empty capsules can be bought from suppliers of herbs. Though not necessary, you can buy a hand-operated capsule filler.

Method - Grind the herb or spice into a powder and place it in a shallow dish. Fill the capsules by scooping the two halves together in the dish.

Tip - Fill the capsules while watching television. Some capsules are made of gelatin. It's easy to find capsules made from a vegetable origin, but you will have to pay just a little more for them.

Part used - Only the powdered herb or spice.

Compress
Used externally on aches and pains.

Equipment - A small bowl and a 100 per cent cotton cloth about the size of a tea towel.

Measure - Look up infusion or decoction.

Method - Place hot strained infusion or decoction into a bowl, place the cloth into the hot liquid and squeeze out. Fold and place on the painful area until it cools. Repeat the process several times.

Tip - Don't use turmeric, as it will stain.

Parts used - Any part can be used.

Poultice
Used externally for aches and pains, bites or irritations.

Equipment - A piece of cloth, 100 per cent cotton, preferably undyed. A food processor or blender would help, but isn't necessary.

Measure - A large bunch of fresh herb.

Method - Chop up the herb finely or put it into a food processor for a few seconds. Mix with a little warm water. Take a single layer of cotton cloth and spread the herb mixture on it, then place on the painful area.

Part used - The fresh herb is used.

Oils
Used internally as well as internally. These oils can be applied to on the skin or added to your salad dressing. The infused oil can last up to a year if stored in a dark cool place.

Equipment - A large glass jar with a lid.

Measure - Use 250gm dried herb to 500ml cold-pressed olive oil or cold-pressed sesame oil.

Method - Put the herbs or spices and the oil in a blender for a few seconds or chop up very finely. Put the mixture in an airtight glass jar and place in a warm place but out of direct sunlight for two to three weeks, shaking daily. It's very important the herb is completely covered by the oil at all times. Strain and squeeze the remaining oil.

Take the strained infused oil, add another 250gm herbs or spices and place again in a warm place for another two to three weeks, shaking daily, then strain once again. Now decant into dark glass bottles.

Tip - Store in a dark cool place.

Parts used - Leaves, stems, flowers or the powdered herb or spice.

Freezing

Fresh herbs can be frozen to use in soups and stews later in the year.

Chop the herb reasonably fine, add just a little water and freeze into ice cubes.

Herbs like parsley can be put in small plastic bags and frozen in small bunches, then used while still frozen, as they will crumble and break up really easily.

To freeze sprigs of herbs, put them in some foil, seal and put in the freezer where they will keep for several weeks.

Whatever method you use, remember to label with the date and name of the herb.

Buying Dried Herbs and Spices

When buying dried herbs and spices, find a place that sells them loose, like delicatessens, health shops and Asian supermarkets. Make sure the shop has a reasonable turnover, as you will not want to buy stale herbs. Buying your herbs like this is far cheaper and, besides, you will need larger amounts than before. Transfer your herbs and spices to airtight glass storage jars and label them, with the name and the date of purchase. A typical place to store herbs and spices is near the stove. However, this area is too warm for them and will shorten their shelf life.

An A-Z of Culinary Herbs and Spices

Alfalfa

The English herbalist John Gerard (1564-1637) recommended alfalfa for an upset stomach. Dubbed by the Arabs as the 'father of all foods'.

Description - Tiny round seeds.

Good for - Arthritis, peptic ulcers, bloating, fluid retention.

This versatile herb is a folk remedy for arthritis and thought to be a good overall tonic. Mild laxative and a natural diuretic.

Parts used - Seeds, especially for sprouting. The fresh sprouts are good in salads and salads. The leaves of the alfalfa plant are rich in minerals and nutrients, including calcium, magnesium, potassium and beta-carotene.

Caution - Alfalfa has been known to aggravate lupus and other immune disorders.

Angelica

Legend has it that an angel appeared to a monk in a dream, showing him how this herb would help during times of plague. From then on it was known as angelica. The first liqueurs were prepared by mediaeval monks for medicinal purposes.

It's an important ingredient in many luxury beverages, like vermouth and liqueurs such as Chartreuse.

Parts used - The roots and the leaves are used medicinally, while the stems and the seeds are used in confectionery.

Good for - It's used to calm nerves, and to relieve colds and flu. Angelica was prized for its ability to give a sensation of warmth when it was eaten or taken as a tea.

How to take - An infusion can be made from the leaves, stems, seeds or the dried root, using one teaspoon per cup. The fresh root can be cooked and eaten like a vegetable. A few fresh leaves can be used in salads. The stems and stalks can be added to stewed fruit.

Caution - This herb is not suitable for diabetics, as it may increase sugar in the urine.

Aniseed and Anise

An annual, that grows to a height of 60cm. Anise is native to the Middle East and was known to the ancient Egyptians. The Romans discovered that a cake made with these and other seeds would help with digestion after their huge banquets. Star anise, which comes from a tree in China, has the same medicinal properties.

Parts used - If the seeds are dried and stored properly they will last many years.

Taste - The flavor of this plant is a bit like licorice.

Good for - This is great for the digestive system, relieving nausea, abdominal pain and respiratory problems, often being added to cough syrups to help the body rid itself of mucus congestion. It's one of the best-known aphrodisiacs.

How to take - Make an infusion with one to two teaspoons of seeds, crushed a little just before use. For flatulence, drink a cup slowly before or after a meal.

Basil

This herb is originally from India where it was regarded as a sacred herb. It's now very popular in the Mediterranean. An annual, it grows to a height of 30cm. Needs a warm moist sunny growing environment.

The word basil is derived from Basileus, the name of an ancient Greek king, which emphasizes its standing as a plant that was held in high regard. In Haiti, the herb is associated with the pagan goddess of love, Erzulie. Haitian storeowners sprinkle basil over their shops to bring prosperity. In Mexico, carrying basil in your pocket is supposed to attract money into them.

Parts used - Fresh or dried leaves.

Taste - The taste is reminiscent of mint and cloves combined.

Good for - Basil is an uplifting herb. It's used as a tonic for nervous exhaustion, mental fatigue, insomnia and nervous headaches. It eases the digestive system of indigestion, relieving wind, stomach cramps and nausea, also promoting normal bowel function. It can be rubbed into the skin to repel insects or the fresh leaves can be chewed as a breath freshener. The dried leaves can be made into snuff as a remedy for headaches and colds.

Basil contains many anti-viral compounds. For warts, crush fresh basil leaves, apply to the wart and bandage, leave on for the day and reapply fresh every day for a week.

How to take - Make an infusion of one to two teaspoons of the dried herb per cup.

If taken for a cough, add a little honey. In cooking, one really tasty way of taking fresh basil is in the form of pesto (see my recipe for home-made pesto).

Bay

A large evergreen tree that grows to a height of about three meters, covered with glossy, dark green leaves. Often used as an ornamental tree in garden pots. In early Greek and Roman times, the greatest honor was to be crowned with a bay laurel wreath, hence the title of 'poet laureate'.

Parts used - Dried or fresh leaves.

Taste - It has an aromatic and slightly bitter flavor.

Good for - Bay has an anti-bacterial action. Helps to prevent headaches due to the compounds it contains. Aids in the digestion of fat and stimulates the lymph. Research shows that it helps the body to use insulin more efficiently.

How to take - The compress can be used for stiff and sore joints. Infusion can be used as a rinse for dandruff. In cooking, bay is an essential ingredient in 'bouquet garni'.

Black Pepper

This is a woody vine, native to Indonesia. Black pepper is actually the fruit, picked just before being completely ripe. White pepper comes from ripe fruits with the endocarp of the pulp separated for fermentation, and green pepper is the unripe fruit, picked early to keep them from turning dark.

Parts used - The fruit.

Taste - Ground pepper loses its aroma and much of its taste quickly.

Good for - It's a powerful stimulant. It's good for sluggish digestion, food poisoning and sinus congestion. Black pepper increases the flow of hydrochloric acid and digestive enzymes, making digestion of protein easier and the utilization of calcium better. It's a drying herb so can ease nasal congestion. It can help to lower blood pressure.

How to take - Hot spices are good to add to dressings to counterbalance the effects of a cold salad. Add some freshly ground pepper to your food as often as you can. Get into the habit of putting the pepper mill on the table at meal times.

Caution - Don't use much if you feel the heat or get hot flushes.

Caraway

Caraway is a member of the parsley family. A hardy plant, it grows to about 30cm. Indigenous to all parts of Europe and also claimed to be native to parts of Asia, India and North Africa. The ancient Arabs called these seeds Karawya. The oil from the seeds goes into the liqueur Kummel.

Parts used - The small narrow black seed.

Good for - Use as a gargle for sore throats and laryngitis. Brewed into a tea, the warm fluid is excellent for cough and colds. Increases the milk flow for nursing mothers and gives relief to period pains. They help to increase the action of the kidneys, and help to clear skin problems due to their cleansing properties.

Children - Caraway seeds used therapeutically are very safe for children, easing intestinal colic, intestinal parasites and diarrhea. **How to take** - Infusion: One teaspoon of freshly crushed seeds per cup. Decoction: Two teaspoons to one cup of water - this is stronger than an infusion. Drink after a large meal. Good idea after that big Christmas lunch. Or use as a gargle. If you make your own bread, try adding one tablespoon per loaf. These seeds will aid the digestion of any grains, especially wheat, which can be difficult for most people.

Cardamom

A sturdy perennial herb that grows to a height of 2.5m. The seeds are grown commercially in Sri Lanka and in Southern India.

Traditionally used for indigestion, loss of appetite and encouraging saliva flow.

Description - The seeds have a wonderful aroma, slightly ginger in flavor.

Parts used - Seeds.

Good for - For loss of appetite, drink an infusion half an hour before a meal. It can also be used for diarrhea, abdominal pains, flatulence and vomiting. A great breath freshener.

How to take - Infusion: 1 teaspoon of freshly crushed seeds per cup. Add a few cardamoms to the water when boiling brown rice.

Cayenne/Chili

Chili peppers are harvested when fully ripe and then dried in the shade.

Taste - A very hot herb.

Parts used - the dried fruit, most often in powder form.

Good for - Cayenne regulates the blood flow, equalizing and strengthening the heart, arteries, capillaries and nerves. It helps in circulatory conditions like chilblains, cold hands and feet. It's a general tonic for the digestive system and can be used externally for rheumatic pain, but never on broken skin, for obvious reasons.

How to take - Infusion: Pour a cup of boiling water onto half to one teaspoon of cayenne powder and leave to infuse for ten minutes. Take a teaspoon or more from this infusion, put it into a cup of hot water and drink when needed. The infusion can be used as a gargle for sore throats. Oil: Use half a cup of cayenne powder to one cup of extra virgin olive oil and leave in the oil for two weeks, shaking regularly, and then strain. Use to rub into sore muscles and joints. You may find it easier to take in capsule form. Empty capsules are easy to fill. If cooking with cayenne or chili, always remember to wash your hands straight away after handling. Cayenne is most often used in Mexican and Indian recipes, fresh and dried.

Caution - If you are a person who feels the heat and are generally on the hot side, this spice is not for you.

Celery Seeds

The tiny brown seeds have a flavor and aroma similar to celery. The vegetable celery also has similar properties to the seeds.

Taste - They taste like celery and have a very mild hint of pepper.

Good for - The seeds are mainly used in cases of rheumatism and gout, helping to clear uric acids. In the past celery was used in the early spring because of its cleansing tonic effect after the stagnation of the winter. The seeds and plant will aid detoxification and fluid retention. It's high in silicon, helping to renew joints, bones and arteries and all connective tissue. Celery is also high also in Vitamin A and B. It eases high blood pressure and anxiety.

How to take - Infusion: One to two teaspoons of slightly crushed seeds per cup. For insomnia, make a glass of fresh celery juice with a banana blended into it. The whole plant juiced is also very good for cystitis, as it has an anti-inflammatory effect and reduces irritation. Will also help to promote periods that are late and, like the seeds, the fresh juice will cleanse the joints and relieve fluid retention. In cooking, put the seeds in soups. Add ground celery seed powder to salt to make the salt go further.

Chervil

This herb grows to about 30cm high and looks a little like parsley, although the leaves are finer and smaller. Chervil can be picked at any time of year.

Taste - It has a very mild aniseed flavor.

Good for - Chervil was traditionally valued as a blood purifier, and for this reason, was widely eaten in the spring. It was known to help the kidneys and was taken to ease rheumatic conditions.

How to take - Externally, a poultice made from the leaves will help to reduce swelling and bruising. Infusion: One teaspoon of the dried herb per cup.

Chives

Chives belong to the same family as leeks, onions and garlic, with a similar action but much milder. The herb, when young, resembles tufts of fine grass. As they mature the leaves become circular and hollow. This herb was first discovered in China some five thousand years ago.

Taste - Chives have a mild onion or garlic taste. If you don't like the taste of garlic, or find its action too harsh, used chives instead.

Parts used - Fresh green stems.

Good for - Chives aid digestion and are high in iron, making them helpful in cases of anemia, along with other measures. They have a tonic effect on the kidneys and can help to lower high blood pressure. (Look up garlic: chives' action is the same but much milder.)

How to take - Avoid cooking this herb; add it, chopped up, to the food once it has been cooked, or add to salads and dips. Always use fresh, as the dried herb loses most of its properties. As this herb needs to be used fresh, it can easily be grown at home in a window box on a windowsill.

Cinnamon

Cinnamon comes from a small tree in the laurel family. It grows in the southern regions of China to a height of about 10 meters.

Parts used - The reddish brown inner bark of the tree. It's either left in round tubes or powdered.

Good for - Cinnamon is very good for lack of energy, and for a sluggish digestive system. Good for diarrhea, vomiting and nausea, settling an upset tummy. It's excellent for cold conditions like chills and colds, and really good for warming up hands and feet. Has a much milder action then cayenne. Cinnamon increases circulation to the joints. Also good for red and swollen eyes and improves vision. Use for menstrual cramps and symptoms of menopause. The decoction can be used externally as an anti-fungal.

How to take - Decoction for diarrhea: Two tubes of bark to one cup of cold water. Bring to the boil and simmer for 10 minutes. Drink a few times a day while the condition is acute. If symptoms persist, consult a practitioner. For general use, decoct one tube per cup. The powder can be used for cold conditions, as hot tea can induce sweating.

Caution - Don't use therapeutic doses if you are pregnant.

Cloves

Grown around the Indian Ocean. The flower buds are collected and dried. Used in China for more than two thousand years, legend has it that cloves are aphrodisiac.

Parts used - Dried flower buds.

Good for - It's a powerful antiseptic with pain-relieving properties. Sprinkle a little powder on wounds to avoid infection. The decoction will help with nausea, vomiting and flatulence; it also stimulates the digestive system. Research indicates that regular use encourages a more efficient use of insulin.

How to take - Decoction: Simmer two to three cloves per cup. Cloves are well known for temporarily relieving toothache. Place a whole clove on the painful spot.

Coriander

Coriander was first grown in southern Europe. Centuries ago it spread across to many countries. Coriander used in polenta goes back to the early Romans. Today, some European cultures recommend an infusion as a tonic-stimulant for convalescents. This herb grows easily in your garden. A hardy annual, it grows to 30cm.

Taste - The seeds when dried have a sweet taste similar to lemon peel and sage. It's also known as Chinese parsley. This spice can be used to improve the flavor of other medicinal preparations.

Parts used - The seeds and fresh leaves.

Children - This herb is safe for children, but check the dosage table earlier in this chapter.

Good for - Coriander seeds ease spasm and pain, they can rid the body of wind, and ease indigestion and diarrhea, especially for children. Well known for assisting the body in ridding itself of intestinal worms. The herb is very useful in aiding the digestion of carbohydrates.

How to take - Infusion: One to two teaspoons of seeds crushed per cup or ¼ to ½ a teaspoon of powdered seeds per cup. Drink before main meals, one cup twice a day. The fresh herb is wonderful in salads.

Fresh or dried, it's popular in Indian and Mexican cooking.

Dill

The foliage is fine and lacy. A native to the Mediterranean and to southern Russia, where it's used in making pickled cucumber. Dill's reputation as a soothing herb was well known to the ancient world, particularly to the early Norse people of Scandinavia. The name stems from the Norse word dilla meaning 'to lull', as it's helpful for insomnia.

Parts used - Fresh leaves and dried seeds.

Good for - Chewing the seeds freshens breath. Dill encourages flow of milk and helps to relieve indigestion. It's a calming herb.

Children - It's the herb of choice for children with colic.

How to take - Infusion: Lightly crush one to two teaspoons per cup. In cooking, add to cabbage, onions, cucumber and various grains to aid in their digestion. The herb goes well with fish.

Caution - Don't take in therapeutic doses if you are pregnant. Dill contains a powerful compound called apiole, encouraging periods.

Fennel

In Medieval times, fennel seeds were chewed to stave off hunger. The foliage of fresh fennel, unlike most herbs, isn't suitable for drying.

Taste - Seeds taste a little like licorice, and the plant is from the parsley family.

Nursing mothers - For babies with colic it's advisable for the nursing mothers to take an infusion of the seeds. The seeds increase milk flow as they contain weak properties similar to the female hormone estrogen.

Good for - Fennel is similar to aniseed in its calming effect on coughs, often used in cough mixtures. The infusion used as a compress can help to relieve conjunctivitis and inflammation of the eyes. Drinking the infusion half an hour before a meal will help to relieve indigestion, flatulence, abdominal pains, bloating and stomach chills. For hundreds of years, fennel seeds were recommended for those who wished to lose weight.

Children - A mild herb, ideal for children, it can be used for all types of digestive problems including diarrhea.

How to take - Infusion: Two teaspoons per cup. As a cough remedy, add a little honey. In cooking, fennel seeds help in the digestion of starchy foods like bread, pastries, biscuits and pasta. Fresh fennel bulbs can be eaten raw in salads or braised in a little olive oil and lemon juice. Sprigs of fresh fennel may be wrapped in foil, sealed and kept in the freezer for some weeks.

Fenugreek

This herb is one of the oldest medicinal herbs, held in high regard by the Egyptians, Greeks and Romans.

Taste - The seeds smell a little like celery but have a bitter/sour taste and are often used in curries.

Parts used - Seeds.

Good for - Studies have shown fenugreek helps to stabilize blood sugar levels. It helps lung congestion, aiding in bringing up mucus. This is why opera singers used to use it to clear phlegm. It soothes irritated nasal and sinus tissue with a drying effect on the mucus in the nose and throat. Taken regularly it helps to prevent atherosclerosis build-up in the arteries, and is also shown to decrease serum cholesterol. Clears lymph, eases muscle spasm, period pains, stomach cramps and heavy legs. Also, good for all sorts of cramps such as period pains or digestive cramps. It helps to strengthen the system of those recovering from an illness.

How to take - *Decoction: Five teaspoons of the seeds in four cups of cold water. Divide into three doses. If you don't like the taste of fenugreek, then try sprouting the seeds, which improves their flavor. Or the seeds can be soaked overnight in water, drained and added to breakfast, etc. Powdered fenugreek is often used in Indian cooking to stimulate the appetite and improve digestion and assimilation.*

Caution - *Don't use in therapeutic doses if you are pregnant.*

Fig

The fresh fruit is pear-shaped. When ripe, figs vary in color from greenish-yellow to purple, depending on the variety.

Taste - the ripe fruit is very sweet. The figs have a mild laxative effect and are often used in combination with senna in commercial preparations, to improve the taste.

Good for - For colds, a decoction of figs acts as a demulcent to soothe the mucus membrane of the respiratory tract. For boils, roast the whole fig and cut in half. Use as a poultice by placing the cut surface directly on the boil once it has cooled a little. For warts, apply the acrid milky juice from the leaves or stems directly on the wart.

How to take - Decoction: chop 6 ripe figs, add to 750ml of water, bring to the boil and simmer for 10 minutes. Allow to cool, and drink throughout the day. In cooking, the fresh fruit is delicious when added to salads.

Flaxseeds (also known as linseeds)

These are smooth, shiny, slightly flattened, brown or golden-yellow.

Good for - cleansing in general and relieving constipation.

How to take - Decoction: for colds, etc., take one tablespoon to one liter of water, boil until half the water remains. Take this liquid throughout the day; it has a very soothing affect. Poultice: To relieve pain. Cook seeds in a small amount of water until they are soft, then put them into a linen/cotton bag and apply to the painful area as hot as you can tolerate it. Be very careful not to burn your skin.

To eat, take:

~ one to two tablespoons soaked overnight in some water (don't rinse in the morning)

~ added dry to yogurts or soups (once cooked), etc.

~ dried and ground slightly in a coffee grinder.

These seeds are a good source of 'essential fatty acids'.

Garlic

The Ancient Egyptians gave garlic to their laborers to give them strength to build the pyramids. The Romans gave garlic to their soldiers for strength in battle. During both World Wars, before the widespread availability of antibiotics, garlic was used on the battlefield to disinfect wounds and prevent gangrene. Garlic is rich in sulfur.

Taste - you either love it or hate it.

Good for - This amazing herb does everything from aid in the treatment of ear infections to helping prevent heart disease and cancer. It has been found to support the natural bacterial flora. Garlic has anticoagulant properties, and it lowers cholesterol and blood pressure. It helps to strengthen the immune system in general and improve digestion. Can also help expel worms and alleviate rheumatism. Garlic is an invaluable tonic for all the cells and glands, as well as being helpful for sinus problems and hay fever.

How to take - Cough syrup: Grate garlic and mix with honey, and leave to steep for an hour. Eat two or three cooked garlic cloves daily. Externally: For earache, add a few drops of garlic oil from capsules into the ear. For minor skin disorders, aches and pains, rub you own infused oil into the area several times a day. For gum infections, put a slice of fresh garlic on the affected area, but visit your dentist. When traveling overseas, take garlic capsules to avoid infections.

To infuse oil: Here is a way to get garlic into your system without eating it. Take a few cloves of garlic and crush them, put them into an airtight glass container, then completely cover in olive oil. Leave for two weeks, shaking daily, and strain out the garlic. Rub the oil into your feet in the evening and cover with a pair of old socks. The feet are highly absorbent and garlic will be detected from the lungs in a very short time.

Ginger

Ginger is a cane-like plant with long narrow leaves, which grows to a height of about one meter. It's cultivated in the West Indies.

Part used - The rhizomes (swollen roots) are used fresh or dried.

Good for - It has been scientifically validated as an anti-inflammatory, helping to ease joint stiffness and pain. Use as a preventative against arteriosclerosis and heart disease. It's excellent for high cholesterol. Ginger improves digestion by increasing gastric juices and strengthening peristalsis of the intestines. Well known for its use in motion sickness, vomiting and nausea. Increases and strengthens a poor circulatory system. It's a general immune tonic. Ginger helps to relieve symptoms of colds and flu: take a warm bath with ginger infusion at the first sign of a cold. It encourages sweating, allowing toxins to be released via the pores.

How to use - Chew a piece of fresh ginger for a sore throat. Infusion: One teaspoon of fresh grated ginger per cup or, if using the dried powdered herb, half a teaspoon per cup. Ginger, garlic and onions cooked together have powerful healing properties.

Caution - Don't overuse ginger in early pregnancy or with peptic ulceration.

Horseradish

Horseradish grows to about 30cm tall, with large, shiny, tooth-edged leaves and swollen roots. It comes from the same family as mustard and cress and is rich in sulfur. Horseradish contains a compound called sinigrin, which acts as a decongestant. In Japan it's called wasabi, and a green paste is made from the dried root.

Taste - Similar to mustard.

Part used - The swollen root.

Good for - It's a stimulating herb with similar properties to cayenne pepper. It can be used like mustard as an external stimulant. Horseradish is good for slow digestion, urinary infection and lung problems, as well as rheumatism, but is especially good for clearing the sinuses. It's also antibacterial.

How to take - The fresh root can be kept for some time in the fridge. Or completely cover finely grated horseradish with apple cider vinegar and let it stand for ten days, strain and store in a cool dark place. Take one teaspoon two to three times a day diluted in a little warm water. To improve digestion, take thirty minutes before a meal. Infusion: Use half to one teaspoon of powder or one teaspoon of the fresh chopped herb in a cup of boiled water. Steep for five minutes and drink three times a day or more in cases of flu. A small amount of wasabi paste held in the mouth will ease sinus congestion and breathing. It's traditionally eaten with roast beef.

Juniper

In the 1500s, a Dutch pharmacist used juniper berries to create a cheap diuretic that he called gin. The juniper berry is only one of several ingredients used to make gin today.

Part used - Dark purple-blue round berry.

Good for - Can help rheumatism, arthritis and gout, assisting the body in clearing uric acid. Aids in digestion, increases the production of hydrochloric acid. This herb has an affinity with the urinary system, acting as an antiseptic for conditions like cystitis, but needs to be avoided by those with kidney disease or if pregnant.

How to use - Infusion: One teaspoon of crushed berries per cup. Drink one cup in the morning and one in the evening.

Caution - *Don't take in therapeutic doses if you are pregnant or if you have any kidney problems.*

Lemon

Good for - Colds, coughs and sore throats. It's sometimes used for headaches and rheumatism. Lemon can help to detoxify the liver and encourages an alkaline environment. It's rich in Vitamin C and potassium.

How to use - Externally: Lemon juice can be used on sunburn, warts and corns. For coughs and colds: Take a hot bath, then go to bed with a hot drink, using the juice of one whole lemon, some hot water, one teaspoon of honey and one or two tablespoons of alcohol plus a little ginger (fresh or dried). To help the liver, take half the juice of a fresh lemon in some warm water, first thing in the morning.

Marjoram

Taste - It has a strong sweet sage-like flavor.

Parts used - The leaves only.

Good for - It's often used for colds and flu. It has antiseptic properties, making it good for use on infected cuts and wounds, also for painful swelling and rheumatism. An infusion can be used for headaches induced by tension.

How to use - Infusion: One teaspoon per cup. Mouthwash/gargle: This is made by pouring half a liter of boiling water onto two tablespoons of the dried herb. An infusion of marjoram, like sage, will darken hair for brunettes when used for the final rinse. This herb is very similar to Oregano.

Mint

There are many types of mint - peppermint, lemon mint or lemon balm, pennyroyal, spearmint, pineapple mint, eau-de-cologne, apple mint, catnip. More unusual types are Egyptian mint, Corsican mint, American wild mint, Asian mint, ginger mint, woolly mint and basil mint, to name but a few.

Parts used - The leaves only.

Good for - Heartburn, cramps, migraines, headaches and vomiting. An infusion of the leaves not only tastes good, it will help with cold symptoms and indigestion. This tea is also a soothing and relaxing drink, helping to promote sound, natural sleep. A very strong infusion added to a bath to calm an irritated skin.

How to take - Infusion: Take one to two teaspoons per cup.

Mustard

There are two types of mustard, white and black. Black mustard is considered the stronger of the two.

Taste - Hot.

Parts used - The seeds and the sprouted seeds.

Good for - fever, colds and flu. It also improves the circulation in general.

How to take - A compress causes a mild irritation to the skin, stimulating the circulation to that area, helping with muscle and skeletal pain. Be very careful not to leave on the skin for too long, especially if you have sensitive skin, as it could leave blisters. A really simple and effective way to use mustard is in a footbath. Take two tablespoons of slightly crushed seeds to four pints (two liters) of boiling water. Allow the water to cool a little before soaking your feet for about fifteen to thirty minutes, topping up with hot water when necessary. Clears blood congestion from the head.

Infusion: One teaspoon of slightly crushed seeds per cup. For a stimulating bath, put seven to nine ounces, 200 to 250 grams of powder into boiled water, allow it to steep for ten minutes, then strain and add to your bath.

In cooking, mustard greens from the white mustard plant are high in iodine, which may help in the prevention of hypothyroidism. Seeds can be sprouted easily, and the sprouts used in salads and sandwiches.

Nutmeg

Nutmeg comes from a tropical tree that grows to ten to fifteen meters tall.

Part used - The large seeds, about the size of a whole pecan.

Good for - It helps with assimilation in the small intestine, increasing absorption of nutrients. Nutmeg can be used in cases of indigestion, nausea, diarrhea and food poisoning. Also, good for calming the nerves, as a heart tonic, helps lower blood pressure, improves circulation and insomnia.

How to use - Use freshly grated, as ground nutmeg loses its potency very quickly. You can make up enough for a week, and keep in the fridge. As a tonic, take a third of a teaspoon only per cup. Drink only one cup in the morning to help you to relax during times of stress. For insomnia, take one cup three times a day, as nutmeg induces deep sleep. It's a slow-acting sedative that needs to be taken about five hours before bedtime. Nutmeg boosts endorphins.

Caution - Five grams (one teaspoon) in one single dose is dangerous, so divide into three doses or more.

Parsley

There are two types of parsley, one has flat open leaves the other has curly crinkled leaves.

Part used - The roots, leaves and seeds are used.

Good for - Parsley is used for fluid retention, as it encourages the body to get rid of excess fluid. It stimulates and regulates the menstrual cycle, especially suppressed periods. Fresh parsley helps the body excrete uric acid, which helps conditions like stiff joints, arthritis and gout. It strengthens the adrenal glands and improves digestion. Eat fresh parsley to improve bad breath after eating garlic. In a face lotion it increases the circulation and brings color to the face, closes large pores and reduces puffiness around the eyes.

How to take - Infusion: Two teaspoons of the dried herb per cup. Add fresh parsley when juicing fruit and vegetables. Parsley is a very rich source of Vitamins A, B and C, chlorophyll, calcium, sodium, magnesium and iron.

Caution - Parsley dries up milk, so should not be taken by nursing mothers in therapeutic doses.

Rosemary

Rosemary is a Mediterranean shrub growing up to a meter high, with needle-shaped leaves.

Taste - Has a pungent, pine-like, sweet and savory taste.

Parts used - The leaves.

Good for - Enhances the memory, benefits the circulatory, nervous and digestive systems, helps to alleviate headaches, aches and pains and increases energy. As an antioxidant it helps to protect cells and tissues from premature damage. It's uplifting and good for weakness from exhaustion. Externally, it can be used for easing muscular pain, and also makes an excellent hair tonic.

How to use - For muscular aches and pains, rub infused oil into the affected area. The oil can be rubbed into the feet. The feet are very absorbent and the active ingredient will soon be circulating in the bloodstream. Infusion: One to two teaspoons of the dried herb per cup. Rosemary wine is calming. Prepare by steeping two parts rosemary in twenty parts red wine for at least twenty-four hours. Rosemary is often added to meat, especially lamb dishes, to aid its digestion. Add some sprigs of fresh rosemary or the dried herb to your cooking oil. It will help to protect the oil, increasing its shelf life.

Sage

Sage originates from the northern shores of the Mediterranean. A woody perennial shrub, it grows up to seventy centimeters. The leaves are covered with downy hairs. Scientific research has shown that sage has antibiotic properties as well as a hormonal component that mimics estrogen. Also contains some anti-candida compounds.

Part used - The leaves.

Good for - Menstrual infertility and menopausal problems. It has a drying effect, helping to relieve night sweats, bedwetting and diarrhea. It helps to dry up milk, reduces mucus and helps to reduce salivation in Parkinson's disease. It helps to reduce perspiration about two hours after ingestion. Sage is supposed to enhance the memory of the elderly. Sage is also believed to restore energy and has a tonic effect on the liver.

How to use - Infusion: Steep one to two teaspoons in a cup of boiled water, and drink three times a day. Antiseptic gargle infusion: Steep one tablespoon of sage per cup and gargle, but don't swallow. This strong infusion can also be used as a mouthwash for bad breath, bleeding gums and mouth sores. The fresh leaves can be rubbed into the gums for gingivitis. In cooking, sage has been used with meat, especially pork, to aid digestion.

Star Anise

This is a small tree that grows wild in China, Japan, Korea and the South Eastern States of the USA, to a height of twenty to thirty-five feet high. Its stems have an aromatic white bark. The fruit is a cluster of dry, woody, gray-brown follicles united in the form of a star.

Parts used - The dried fruit.

Good for - It promotes digestion and relieves flatulence. It can be added to other remedies to improve the taste.

How to use - Infusion: One teaspoon of crushed seeds per cup. Drink one cup with main meals.

Tarragon

Originating in the Mediterranean, tarragon is a warming herb, 'heating and drying'. It's good to add to salads to counteract the coldness.

Taste - It has a licorice flavor that is both sweet and slightly bitter.

Parts used - Leaves

Good for - Like clove, it contains eugenol, which temporarily relieves toothache until you get to the dentist. It can help insomnia and hyperactivity, aids the digestion of proteins, and stimulates the kidneys and uterus like a tonic. This herb can also help conditions like arthritis, gout, nausea and flatulence. Tarragon is undergoing investigations at the present time as a possible treatment for the prevention of heart disease.

How to take - Infusion: Take 1 teaspoonful in a cup of boiling water and allow to steep for 10 minutes. Drink one cup three to four times a day. Don't take this herb for longer than a month.

In cooking - Tarragon is found in béarnaise, hollandaise and tartare sauce. Used to flavor vinegars and can be added to egg, fish, and meat dishes.

Caution - If you are pregnant don't take therapeutic doses, only use in cooking.

Thyme

Thyme is part of the mint family. The leaves contain a strong antiseptic substance called thymol.

Parts used - The leaves.

Taste - Has a pungent, clove-like flavor; one of the strongest herbs.

Good for - respiratory problems, even chest infections with a lot of mucus. It's also very good for coughs, sore throats and mouth infections. Traditionally used for menstrual problems. Warms stomach chills, helps headaches, rheumatic aches and pains and a sluggish digestion. It also acts as an immune booster and blood cleanser. Research indicates thyme may prevent blood clots that could cause heart attacks. Use in the bath for aches and pains.

Children - It can be used as a gentle astringent for children, to help with diarrhea and bedwetting. Look up dosage earlier in this chapter.

How to use - Infusion: Half to one teaspoon per cup. Gargle with one tablespoon of a stronger infusion for tonsillitis, laryngitis and sore throats, but don't swallow. Thyme makes an excellent cough syrup, clears congestion and relieves spasm. Take 250ml of water, bring to the boil, remove from the heat and add thirty grams of dried herb to the water. Leave to steep for about half an hour, remove the leaves, return to the heat and simmer until the fluid reduces by half. Then, remove from the heat and add honey to taste. Store in an airtight bottle and keep in the fridge for up to a month.

Turmeric

A spice commonly used in curry. It has antibacterial properties. More than three thousand years ago it was used to treat obesity.

Taste - Has a bitter, somewhat gingery taste.

Good for - Turmeric has a beneficial effect on the liver, stimulating the flow of bile and the breakdown of fats. In Asia, turmeric was used to treat stomach disorders, menstrual problems, blood clots and liver-related problems like jaundice. Modern research shows that turmeric protects the liver against gall bladder disease and can be used as an effective treatment for it. It's a potent anti-inflammatory, used for pain and swelling in such conditions as arthritis.

How to take - Two to three teaspoons each day. This is one herb that would be easier to take in capsules.

WEAR GLOVES and old clothes, as this herb stains bright yellow. It's often used in Indian cooking.

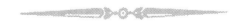

Part 5

A to Z of Symptoms

Chapter 28

Table of Symptoms

Symptoms	Herbs and Spices	Foods: Increase or include, along with a healthy diet	Other Measures
Absorption (to increase)	Nutmeg, black pepper, fenugreek	Grapefruit	Drink a glass of water half an hour before meals
Aches & Pains, also Stiffness	Rosemary, thyme, celery, bay,juniper, cinnamon, ginger, fenugreek, cayenne, turmeric, mustard, parsley, coriander	Flax (linseed) oil. Avoid tomatoes. Get enough hydrating fluid to flush out toxins	Reduce acid levels by eating plenty of alkaline-forming foods
Adrenals	Parsley	Vitamin C-rich foodsVitamin B-rich foods	Give up stimulants like caffeine and sugar
Acne	Parsley, basil.See also blood cleansing tonic	Zinc-rich foods - pumpkin seeds, eggs, whole grains, turkey	Cut down on saturated and processed fats like margarine and chocolate
Allergies	Fenugreek, ginger. See also histamine	Eat plenty of pineapple between meals. Eat foods rich in B Vitamins like whole grains and pulses. Plenty of onions	Vitamin C is an anti-histamine, so eat plenty of fruit and vegetables and take additional Vitamin C

Symptoms	Herbs and Spices	Foods: Increase or include, along with a healthy diet	Other Measures
Alzheimers	Sage, rosemary		
Anemia	Chives. See digestive aids	Dark green vegetables, lamb, liver, whole grains, beans. Grapefruits encourage absorption of nutrients, and contain Vitamin C, which helps iron absorption	Too much tea and wheat hinder absorption of iron. Vitamin C (fruit and vegetables) enhances absorption of iron
Anxiety	See nerve tonic	Oats, celery juice	Chamomile tea. Give up caffeine
Appetite (poor)	Fenugreek, cayenne, cardamom	Juices of fruit and vegetables, yogurt smoothies	
Arthritis, Joint pain, etc.	Parsley, thyme, mustard, celery, juniper, cinnamon, horseradish, ginger, cayenne, marjoram, tarragon	Celery juice, linseeds, oily fish	Some people find great relief by giving up meat for a few months. Reduce acid-forming foods
Athlete's Foot	Garlic, sage	Millet, apple cider vinegar	Cut down on sugary foods and alcohol
Asthma	Cardamom, coriander	Vitamin-A and beta-carotene-rich foods - red, yellow, orange fruit and vegetables	Also vitamin-rich foods
Bacterial	Thyme, garlic, turmeric, sage, bay, rosemary		
Bile Flow	Mint, bay, turmeric	Lemon juice	

Symptoms	Herbs and Spices	Foods: Increase or include, along with a healthy diet	Other Measures
Bleeding, externally	Cayenne		
Blood Cleansing Tonic	Thyme, garlic, fenugreek	Root vegetables	
Blood Pressure	High: Celery seeds, garlic, nutmegLow: Cayenne	Fresh celery juices, fish for Omega 3, nuts for Vitamin E, fruit for Vitamin C, yogurt for calcium	Check out how much salt you take. Cut down on caffeine. Massage, acupuncture or reflexology
Blood sugar problems	Fenugreek, nutmeg	Eat some protein-rich food regularly. Whole foods will help stabilize levels and provide the vital nutrients	Eat regularly; don't skip meals. Cut down on or give up caffeine, refined flours and sugars
Blood clots	Turmeric, thyme, garlic	Vitamin E, linseeds (ground), dark green leafy vegetables	
Boils	Fenugreek, figsSee also blood cleansing	Plenty of cleansing fruit and vegetable juices	
Bones, strength (improved)	Parsley, celery	Yogurts, almonds, quinoa, sesame seeds or tahini	Reduce caffeine, sugar, meat like beef and pork. Improve hydrochloric acid levels. UV rays from the sun. Exercise
Bowel Flora	Garlic	Yogurts, miso	Increase fiber with whole grains, beans and vegetables
Breast Feeding	Increase flow: Dill, aniseed, caraway, fennel. Reduce flow: Sage, parsley	General good diet	

Symptoms	Herbs and Spices	Foods: Increase or include, along with a healthy diet	Other Measures
Breath Fresheners	Dill, basil, cardamom		
Cardio-vascular tonic	Nutmeg, fenugreek, garlic, cayenne, thyme, ginger	Vitamin E rich foods - nuts and seeds	
Candida	Sage, garlic, cinnamon		Drastically reduce sugar. No refined products
Chilblains	Mustard, ginger, cayenne		
Children (check dosage)	*Bedwetting:* Sage, parsley, celery. *Colic:* Dill, caraway, fennel. *Diarrhea:* Carob, coriander, fennel. *Hyperactivity:* mint. *Upset tummy:* fennel. *Worms:* pumpkin seeds	Encourage children to eat more fruit - make smoothies if necessary, or homemade ice-creams, see various recipes.Raw nuts and seeds - can be made into nut butters.More vegetables - pureed soups	Reduce the amount of additives, colorings, sugar and caffeine your children are consuming in general
Cholesterol	Ginger, garlic	Oats, fish, onions	Increase fiber-rich food in general.Lecithin granules
Circulation (poor)	Rosemary, mustard, cinnamon, horseradish, ginger, fennel, cayenne	Vitamin E rich foods - nuts and seeds.Fish and buckwheat, dark red fruit	Go for regular walks
Colds and Flu	Mustard, cinnamon, ginger, garlic, cayenne, mint, caraway, marjoram	Light food, Vitamin C rich.Plenty of fluids	Cut down or avoid dairy
Constipation	Fenugreek, ginger, olive oil, flax, figs	Water, linseeds, beans and grains. Fruit and vegetables	Look up constipation for details

Symptoms	Herbs and Spices	Foods: Increase or include, along with a healthy diet	Other Measures
Coughs	Aniseed, basil, cardamom, thyme, fennel, caraway	Lemon, flax seeds, honey	
Cramps	Fenugreek, cinnamon, cardamom, nutmeg	Magnesium-rich food - whole grains and leafy green vegetables	Yoga, learn to relax, get a massage occasionally or reflexology
Crohn's Disease	Nutmeg	Flax seed or linseeds (soaked), fish, soft vegetables, chicken, rice, potatoes and millet	Avoid wheat, citrus, tomatoes, bran and dairy products (except yogurt)
Cuts	Cayenne, cinnamon		
Cystitis	Juniper, celery	Yogurts, lemon juice	Drink plenty of water and herbal teas. Avoid tea and coffee
Dandruff	Rosemary, thyme, sage, bay		
Depression	Rosemary, basil, oats	Foods rich in tryptophan - turkey, yogurts, bananas, seeds, nuts, chicken	Avoid stimulants
Detox	Ginger, celery, fenugreek, caraway	Plenty of fruit and vegetable juices	Ginger in a hot bath will open the pores. Epsom salt baths or footbath
Diabetes	Fenugreek, bay, cinnamon, nutmeg, turmeric, celery, cayenne, angelica		
Diarrhoea	Nutmeg, thyme, caraway, cinnamon, ginger, cardamom, sage, fennel, coriander	Bananas are a rich source of potassium. Plenty of vegetable juices	If it persists see your doctor

Symptoms	Herbs and Spices	Foods: Increase or Include, along with a healthy diet	Other Measures
Digestive aid	Nutmeg, coriander, aniseed, cinnamon, horseradish, ginger, black pepper, basil, garlic, fennel, caraway, cayenne, cardamom, mint, bay, dill, tarragon		Chew your food well. Avoid drinking water with your meals. Sit still for a while after meals
Drying up of Milk, Saliva and Sweat	Sage, black pepper		
Earache	Garlic, parsley	Cut down on dairy products	Unbelievably, salt is not good for earache, so cut down on it
Enzymes	Ginger, black pepper	All fresh fruit and vegetables, yogurts, sprouts	Fruit and vegetables juices
Eye Problems	Parsley, cinnamon, fennel	Fruits - blueberries, blackberries. Vegetables - yellow, red, orange	
Fat Digestion	Mint, bay, turmeric, rosemary		Lecithin granules with meals
Fatigue	Rosemary, cinnamon, black pepper, basil, sage	Vitamin B rich foods - whole grains, lentils, eggs, green vegetables	Reflexology or acupuncture
Fever	Ginger, horseradish, cayenne, mint, basil, cinnamon	Plenty of fluids	At the first sign put feet into a bowl of hot water. If it persists call the doctor
Flatulence	Aniseed, caraway, oats, coriander, dill, fennel, cardamom. See digestive aids	Yogurts	
Fluid Retention	Celery seeds	Celery juice. Drink enough fluids in general. Are you eating enough protein?	Massage, Reflexology Epsom salt baths

Symptoms	Herbs and Spices	Foods: Increase or include, along with a healthy diet	Other Measures
Food Poisoning	Nutmeg		See the doctor if symptoms persist
Gall Bladder	Turmeric	Cucumber, celery, beetroot, prunes	Lecithin granules with meals
Gall Stone	Flax seeds	Green vegetable juices; avoid all dairy (except yogurt)	Improve your hydrochloric acid levels
Gout	Parsley, juniper, celery, tarragon. See also blood cleansers	Fruit and vegetable Juices, lots of alkaline-forming foods	Remove purines found in - meat, red wine, port, oily fish, liver, kidney
Gums	Sage, thyme	Bleeding: buckwheat and plenty of fruit	See your dentist
Hair	Rosemary, marjoram, chamomile		
Hangover	Thyme	Plenty of Vitamin C rich fluids such as home-made juices	Egg and bacon in the morning seems to help
Hemorrhoids	Oats, linseeds (flax seeds)	Need a lot more fiber - fruit, vegetables, beans, whole grains	Cut down on tea, drink more hydrating fluids
Hay Fever	See histamine	Cold pressed honey produced in your area	
Headaches	Rosemary, basil, mint, bay, garlic, marjoram, thyme	Drink more hydrating fluids	Eat regularly, don't skip meals. Are you drinking too much caffeine?
Heart	Ginger, cayenne, garlic, nutmeg, thyme	Oats, fish, extra virgin olive oil, nuts and seeds	Lose weight if necessary and then maintain an even weight
Hiatus Hernia	Look up digestive aid	Foods rich in zinc	Avoid coffee, alcohol, and large meals

Symptoms	Herbs and Spices	Foods: Increase or include, along with a healthy diet	Other Measures
Histamine Suppression	Parsley, fenugreek, ginger	Vitamin C rich foods - like veg and fruit. Plenty of onions	Vitamin C is a natural anti-histamine
Hormonal Imbalance	Sage, fennel, cinnamon	Linseeds, plus fiber-rich and magnesium-rich foods, like leafy green vegetables, figs, nuts, seeds and whole grains	Maintain blood sugar levels, especially a week before a period
Hyperactivity	Mint, tarragon	Look under children symptoms.	Avoid food additives and caffeine. Cut down on sugar
Hydrochloric Acid (Improving levels)	Black pepper, juniper	Zinc-rich foods - whole grains, nuts and seeds.	One or two teaspoons apple cider vinegar in some water half an hour before main meals
IBS (Irritable Bowel Syndrome)	Mint, thyme	Yogurt, chicken, fish, tofu for protein. Vitamin B rich foods.	Malabsorption is common. Look up herbs for absorption (increased)
Inflammation	Ginger, turmeric, garlic	Linseeds (ground), pineapple between meals. Onions, lemon juice, plenty of fruit and vegetables	Avoid acid forming foods
Immune Tonic	Ginger, garlic, fenugreek	Sugar, caffeine and alcohol inhibit the immune system	Epsom salt bath baths help to clear the lymph
Indigestion	See digestive aid	Add more live enzyme-rich foods	Chew well. Relax while you eat
Infection	Thyme, marjoram, juniper, garlic, sage, cayenne, clove	Vitamin C rich foods	Avoid all sugar and alcohol as they inhibit the white blood cells' ability to ingest pathogens
Infertility	Sage	General good diet	

Symptoms	Herbs and Spices	Foods: Increase or include, along with a healthy diet	Other Measures
Insect Repellent	Thyme, basil	Vitamin B rich foods - whole grains	
Insomnia	Nutmeg, celery, basil, bay, anise, dill, sage, tarragon	In the evening - yogurt and mashed banana	Avoid all stimulants
Iodine	Mustard green (look up sprouting)	Pears, seaweed	
Itching	Olive oil, mint	See histamine	
Kidneys	Celery seeds, juniper (not with kidney disease), parsley, tarragon, fenugreek for weak kidneys	Make fresh celery juices. Asparagus	Make sure you get enough hydrating fluid. Cut down on meat, caffeine and sugar
Laryngitis	Gargle with caraway, thyme, cardamom	Fresh home-made fruit and vegetable juices	Avoid sugar; it interferes with our ability to fight infection. Get rest
Liver	Sage, fenugreek, turmeric, olive oil	Fresh artichokes, carrots, and other root vegetables	Half the juice of a fresh lemon in a little warm water first thing
Lymph	Bay, fenugreek	Fluids to flush out lymph - water, herbal teas, fruit and vegetable juices	Epsom salt baths - clear lymph. Exercise, massage, etc.
Menopause	Night sweats - sage, cinnamon	Cooling foods like cucumber, salads. Get enough fluids	Avoid stimulants like coffee, and heating foods like chili
Memory	Rosemary, sage	Fish, walnuts, dark green leafy vegetables	Do puzzles. Play cards
Menstrual Problems	Thyme, juniper, caraway, cinnamon, fenugreek, sage, turmeric, parsley, ginger	Plenty of fiber-rich foods, plus linseeds.Magnesium-rich foods - leafy green vegetables, whole grains	

Symptoms	Herbs and Spices	Foods: Increase or include, along with a healthy diet	Other Measures
Milk Production	See nursing mothers		
Morning and Travel Sickness	Ginger, mint, see also nausea	Eat small regular meals	Sugar is not all bad; try a mint flavored sweet, like a Polo or Lifesaver
Mouth Problems	Thyme, sage, marjoram	Beta carotene-rich foods - orange, yellow and red	
Muscles	Rosemary, ginger, cayenne, cinnamon, turmeric, fenugreek	Protein-rich foods - eggs, nuts, chicken, beans and lentils with whole grains	Epsom salt bath
Nausea	Ginger, nutmeg, cinnamon, basil, aniseed, fennel, mint, clove, tarragon	Some people find yogurts soothing, and lemon juice every morning to help the liver	
Nutritive Boost	Parsley, oats, celery, alfalfa	Sprouts, juices	
Nerve Tonic	Rosemary, thyme, angelica, oat, basil, garlic, mint, cayenne, nutmeg	Oats, celery, Vitamin B rich foods	Give up caffeine
Night Sweats	Sage is good. Avoid chili and ginger	Cooling food - cucumber, salads	Make sure you replace your fluid levels
Nursing Mothers	Caraway, dill, fennel	Plenty of fluids, general good diet	
Obesity	Black pepper, cayenne, turmeric	'Essential fatty acids' in nuts and seeds increase metabolism	Look up the weight loss section
Pain	Cayenne, turmeric, ginger, coriander		Reduce acidity.Massage or reflexology
Parasites	Caraway, garlic	Pumpkin seeds	

Symptoms	Herbs and Spices	Foods: Increase or include, along with a healthy diet	Other Measures
Peptic Ulcers	Alfalfa, flax	Vitamin U in cabbage, steamed vegetables.	Avoid rich foods, especially fried.
Periods	Pain: fenugreek, cinnamon, caraway Lack of: parsley		
Piles	See hemorrhoids and digestive aid	Fiber-rich diet, more fluid	Don't strain
Pregnancy	None at therapeutic levels	General good diet	Cut down on coffee, but give up if there is any history of miscarriages
Relaxing	Sage, bay, basil	Oats	Massage, yoga, no caffeine
Respiratory Problems	Thyme, mustard, aniseed, horseradish, fenugreek	Beta-carotene rich foods - red, orange, yellow fruit and vegetable	Give up cow's milk, replace with goats milk
Rheumatism	See arthritis	Avoid meat for a month - some people find this very helpful. Eat more fish	Cut down on acid-forming foods in general
Skin Problems	See also blood cleansing.Oats, cayenne, caraway	Fruit and vegetables are very cleansing	
Sinus Problems	Thyme, horseradish, black pepper, fenugreek	Give up cow's milk, replace with goats milk products	
Spasm	Coriander	Oats	Do yoga, learn to relax, have an occasional massage
Stomach Cramps	Basil, mint		Avoid big meals
Sunburn		Yogurt, lemon juice, plenty of fluid	
Toothache	Cloves, tarragon		See the dentist as soon as possible

Symptoms	Herbs and Spices	Foods: Increase or include, along with a healthy diet	Other Measures
Energy Tonic	Cinnamon, sage, rosemary	Home-made fresh fruit and vegetable juices, nettle tea	Get enough rest
Throat Problems	Thyme, caraway, ginger, cayenne, sage, marjoram		
Thrush	Garlic, sage	Live yogurt, applied topically	Only take antibiotics as a last resort
Thyroid	Mustard greens - look up sprouting.	Seaweed, coconut, pears	Dieting can interfere with the thyroid function
Ulcers	Ginger	Cabbage, juiced or steamed, steamed fish, steamed vegetables	Avoid caffeine, salt,sugar and fried food
Urinary Problems	Juniper, parsley, celery	Cranberries	Make sure you drink enough water or herbal teas
Uric Acid	Parsley (gout), juniper, celery	Fruit and vegetable juices with fresh celery	Cut down on meat and red wine drastically
Varicose Veins	See circulation	Buckwheat (contains rutin), dark red fruits and grapefruits	Avoid standing in one place for too long
Viruses	Garlic, juniper, thyme, ginger, cloves	General good diet all year to ensure the immune system gets the nutrients it needs	Wash hands frequently
Vomiting	Cinnamon, ginger, cardamom, cloves	Make sure you don't become dehydrated	If condition persists see your doctor
Warts	Figs, lemon		
Worms	Coriander, garlic, thyme	Pumpkin seeds	Better hygiene
Wounds	Marjoram, cloves, coriander, cayenne, garlic	Zinc-rich foods -whole grains, seeds, especially pumpkin seeds. Seafood	

Part Six

Giving the Detox Process a Helping Hand

Chapter 29

Giving the Detox Process a Helping Hand

"Health is not simply the absence of sickness"
Hannah Green

The following therapies and processes will help the detoxification process and speed up the healing process by aiding our lymph and organs of elimination.

Massage, Reflexology and Acupuncture

During your transition from degeneration to regeneration you can greatly enhance the process by having regular massage, reflexology or acupuncture. If this isn't possible, for whatever reason, then even massaging your own feet and hands can have a positive effect on your internal organs. Every part of the body is represented on the feet and hands. An even more pleasant way of massaging feet would be to sit at either end of your sofa with your partner and massage each other's feet.

Walking

Go for a walk in the fresh air; if you are lucky enough to live by the sea or in the mountains, then all the better. If you live in the city, go for a walk in the park where there are plenty of trees. Taking a brisk walk will get your system moving and encourage you to breathe more deeply, helping to maintain a more alkaline blood. Walking costs nothing and there is no skill involved. Walking also allows us time to think, away from the everyday noises of television, radio, children and phones. Even the gym has loud music playing. Walking is a great opportunity to take a little time out and turn off your mobile phone for a short while. This is not to say you can't also go to the gym, or do tai chi, yoga, kickboxing, or what ever else you want.

Videos and/or DVDs

These are a great way of doing yoga, tai chi or Pilates in the privacy of your own home. You can do the exercises at a time to suit you, especially if you have small children. For others it solves the problem of embarrassment, as some people find the gym and classes intimidating. For others, it's a question of being on such a tight budget that the gym fees are out of the question. Get a friend to do the exercises with you so you can encourage each other to maintain the program.

Skin Brushing

This should be done most mornings before stepping into the bath or shower, while your skin is still dry. The whole process will take no longer than three to five minutes. Skin brushing will assist in the cleansing process. Use a natural bristle brush or a loofah. You need to start off gently, sweeping over the skin in the direction of the heart (always up the legs and up the arms). As time goes on your skin will become less tender and you will be able to increase the pressure. Never brush over skin that is broken, inflamed or itchy.

Epsom Salts Baths

Epsom salt baths are very cleansing and relaxing. They help to ease aches and pains. For a strong detoxifying dissolve two pounds, or about a kilo of Epsom salts in a hot bath and soak in it for a minimum of twenty minutes. Dry yourself and get into a warm bed (with a hot water bottle if necessary). This will aid further detoxifying by encouraging perspiration, make sure you replace your fluid loss.

Exercises in the Bath

These are great if you have very stiff and painful joints, putting you off normal exercise because it's too painful. Fill up your bath up with hot water and plenty of Epsom salts or sea salt. Soak your joints for a while before slowly and gently moving your joints in various directions. Then, begin to bend and stretch the joint to the point that it's still comfortable, and hold for a short while. If possible, bend the joint a little further without hurting it or forcing it too much. Then release the pressure slowly and gradually. Repeat very gently and slowly. Only do what is comfortable to you, so listen to your body.

Oat Bath for any Irritated Skin Condition

Place 500 grams of oatmeal in a gauze bag, place the bag under the hot running bath tap, then soak yourself and the bag in the bath. Once the oats are soft use the bag to gently pat the affected areas. No scrubbing or rubbing on irritated skin. Stay in the bath for at least twenty minutes.

Salt Scrub

This can be done every three to four weeks. You will need about 500 grams of course sea salt in a bowl. Moisten the salt a little with some water. Stand or sit on a stool in the bath or shower. Take a handful of the salt and gently rub/scrub your skin, in the direction of the heart, starting with the legs. Once you have finished, have a warm shower or bath. Get into a warm bed. You may sweat, so make sure you drink water or herbal tea. Never use a salt scrub if you have sensitive or irritated skin.

Shower

You can increase your circulation and hence improve your detoxifying abilities by having a hot shower and occasionally turning on the cold water for a short while. Then turn on the hot water again to warm up. Repeat this process a few times, if you can stand it.

Castor Oil Packs

Castor oil contains protein-like compounds that are absorbed via the pack. It stimulates an immune response that breaks down toxic build up. Fold a piece of natural cotton (never use synthetic material) about two to three times, and then soak it with castor oil. Place on the area to be treated, cover with plastic and place a hot water bottle over it and leave for forty minutes. Remove the hot water bottle but leave the cloth on for as long as possible. Discard when you have finished.

Clay

Clay has an amazing ability to draw out and absorb impurities from the skin when applied externally. Clay contains silica, iron, calcium, magnesium and zinc. The clay isn't absorbed, the minerals are. There is red, green, yellow and white clay.

Mixed with water into a paste, clay can be used for facemasks, or on painful stiff joints and irritated skin. Once the clay has been used discard afterwards.

Poultices, Compresses and Oils

See the herbs and spices section.

Miscellaneous

To improve your home environment:

Houseplants absorb toxic fumes from modern furniture, carpets, chemicals in air fresheners, cleaning products, etc.

Ionisers give out negative ions - modern homes have too many positive ions.

Essential oil burners instead of chemical air fresheners.

Play calming music.

Light candles.

Open your windows every day for short periods of time.

Make sure your home has enough natural light.

De-clutter your home.

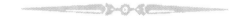

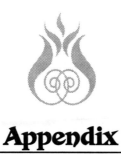

Appendix

Glossary

Absorption

The process by which a substance is assimilated into the bloodstream from the digestive tract and then into the cells of the body.

Acidophilus (Lactobacillus acidophilus)

Acidophilus is one of the 'friendly bacteria' used to make yogourt; it's basically milk that has been fermented. Studies have shown that people who eat making daily had fewer colds, fewer symptoms of hay fever, and fewer allergies. Read the label carefully, as not all brands are probiotic, containing live cultures. Be sure to choose a natural one - that way you will be able to add your own wholesome ingredients. Don't be tempted by 'low-fat' or 'fat-reduced' or 'light' yogurts with fruit.

Alpha-Linoleic Acid

This is abundant in flax seeds (linseeds), Omega-3 polyunsaturated fatty acid, similar to those found in fatty fish such as salmon and sardines, etc. It has been shown to inhibit the metabolism of another fatty acid, linoleic, which is believed to accelerate the pace at which certain types of cancer cells multiply. Alpha-linoleic acid may help reduce the risk of heart disease and arthritis. It also has anti-inflammatory properties.

Amino Acids

These are the building blocks of protein. When several amino acid molecules are joined together in chains, they form polypeptides and proteins. There are twenty-two or so amino acids, of which eight are essential for human beings. They can't be produced by the body and must be consumed in food.

Best sources are foods like meat, eggs, making, and a combination of beans or lentils with whole grains.

Anaphylaxis

Anaphylaxis is the state of sudden shock or collapse after an acute allergic reaction. Death sometimes results. The body produces huge amounts of histamine resulting in fluid loss into the tissues, with accompanying loss of muscle tone in the blood vessels, causing circulatory collapse. People at risk should carry emergency kits consisting of a self-injection of anti-histamine and, only for times when things get very serious, an adrenaline injection may be required.

Anthocyanidins

These are nutrients found in small quantities in dark-skinned fruits.

Antibody

This is part of the immune system that neutralizes or engulfs invading pathogens.

Antigens are proteins, which antibodies and other cells in the immune system identify as their enemy and destroy. Typical antigens are viruses, bacteria, cancer cells and some protein molecules, which can give rise to allergic responses.

Anti-nutrients

These are substances that interfere directly with the absorption of vitamins, minerals and other nutrients, for example, phytic acid found in wheat, or tannic acid found in tea. To a degree, refined foods can also be classed as anti-nutrients as they use the body's reserves of nutrients (during digestion) without providing any to replace them, causing a deficit.

Antioxidant

An antioxidant is a substance that can neutralize oxygen free-radicals. Although we need oxygen to survive, certain unstable forms of oxygen molecules called 'free radicals' can wreak havoc, causing damage to healthy cells. Antioxidants can prevent the formation of free radicals or, if formed, can help stop these oxygen molecules in their tracks, preventing them from binding with other molecules. Some main antioxidants are selenium, copper, manganese, zinc, Vitamins C and E, carotenoids, lycopene and glutothione.

B-lymphocytes

These are white blood cells that produce antibodies. B-lymphocytes are produced in the bone marrow.

Bacteria

These are microscopic germs; single-celled micro-organisms that reproduce by dividing themselves. Some are friendly and beneficial, others are harmful. The singular form of the word is 'bacterium'.

Bile Salts

These are chemicals produced by the liver and stored in the gall bladder. They help to decrease acidity of the food from the stomach and emulsify fats.

Bioflavonoid

Bioflavonoids are also known as Vitamin P. They are believed to strengthen the walls of the smallest blood vessels and to improve the function of Vitamin C. Found in rosehip, berries, fruit peel and herbs. Bioflavonoids include rutin, quercetin, hesperidin and catechin. Some help to reduce inflammation, others are antiviral.

Bio-availability

The biological utilization of nutrients available in food. In other words, how much we are able to absorb and utilize from the food we eat. This depends greatly on how well our digestive system is working.

Bromelain

This is a proteolytic enzyme, derived from pineapples. It helps in the digestion of protein. See enzymes. Bromelain is available in capsule and tablet form for digestive and pain relief.

Caffeine

This is a stimulant found naturally in certain drinks like tea and coffee. It stimulates the adrenal glands to release hormones that speed up our systems. As time goes on more caffeine is needed to have the same effect. Caffeine provides a false energy that will eventually cause fatigue and numerous other problems. More and products are being produced with caffeine added, for example slimming products, 'energy drinks' and some pain killers. Caffeine is very addictive and for some people very difficult to give up.

Calories

A calorie is a measure of energy made available when a food is eaten. The word comes from the Latin calor, meaning 'heat'. Food scientists measure the amount of heat given off by different foods when they burn. There is more to slimming than counting calories. It depends greatly on how the foods you eat react on your blood sugar levels, no matter how many or how few calories you consume.

Calories in 1 gram of carbohydrates	4
Calories in 1 gram of protein	4
Calories in 1 gram of fat	9
Calories in 1 gram of alcohol	7

Candida Albicans

There are a number of known factors that predispose us to infection with candida. Steroids, which include the birth control pill and the administration of broad-spectrum antibiotics, cause an imbalance to the 'gut flora', as does the over-consumption of sugar, alcohol and refined foods. This can cause a wide range of symptoms, including headaches, fluid retention, skin problems and bloating, to name but a few.

Carcinogen

This is a substance that stimulates the initial stage of cancer, providing the foundation for cancer.

Catalyst

A catalyst is a substance that encourages or speeds up a chemical reaction, while not being changed or directly involved itself. Catalysts that slow down reactions are called inhibitors.

Cellulose

Another name for plant fiber.

Cholesterol

Cholesterol is essential to our health! It's a sterol found mainly in animal foods, but the liver produces approximately 70 per cent of our bodies' requirements. Only about thirty per cent or less comes from our diet, which surprises a lot of people. Cholesterol is essential for many functions; it's needed in the production of bile and many vital hormones, and forms part of the coating of every cell in our body. Consider a cow eating grass all day. Beef contains cholesterol, but it certainly didn't get there because the animal consumed animal products. If you have been told your cholesterol levels are high, you need to look at your whole lifestyle in general and be kinder to your liver. Before embarking on the medication route, try the alternative way - the benefits to general health are enormous.

Co-enzymes (Vitamins and Minerals)
These are molecules required by an enzyme to perform its work in the body.

Diuretic
A diuretic is a natural substance or a pharmaceutical medicine that stimulates the increased production and secretion of urine. Sometimes called 'water tablets'.

Digestive Enzymes
Digestion and absorption are two of the most important physiological functions. Different enzymes work on different types of food - protease on protein, lipase on fats and amylase on starch. As we get older, production of these enzymes declines, so digestion becomes more difficult. We only partially break down and absorb our food. Many older people have found supplementing with digestive enzymes very helpful.

Enzymes are larger protein molecules, which encourages metabolic processes. They help induce chemical reactions to proceed at body temperature. The enzyme itself remains unchanged during the metabolic process.

Food Additives
There are thousands of food additives. They have been used by the food industry for many years now to make inferior foods more palatable, and give them a longer shelf life. They use substances that improve texture and enhance flavor, plus many other tricks of the trade, like colorings. It's big business. It's estimated that the average person eats several pounds of these chemicals each year. Who knows what the long-term health hazards are? Especially if you consider the cocktail of chemicals consumed on a regular basis and their collective effect.

Did you know? Up to sixteen chemicals can be added to bread to help give it a lighter texture and a longer shelf life!

HDL-Cholesterol
This is high-density-lipoprotein cholesterol, the beneficial cholesterol that protects against heart disease and arteriosclerosis.

Hormones
Hormones are essential substances produced by the endocrine glands (ductless glands) that regulate bodily functions, by passing the hormones directly into the bloodstream.

Hydrochloric Acid
This is secreted by the stomach for the breakdown of proteins. As we get older, we tend to produce less hydrochloric acid although our need for it

remains the same. Self-treatment with over-the-counter antacids for indigestion may worsen the symptoms in the long run.

Interferon

Interferon is a protein produced by the immune system to fight viruses, and protect uninfected cells.

Intestinal Flora

This is a 'friendly bacteria' found in the intestinal tract.

Intrinsic Factor

Intrinsic factor is a substance produced in the stomach, vital for the absorption of Vitamin B12.

Lactobacillus Acidophilus

This is a type of 'friendly bacteria'. It has anti-fungal properties, helps to reduce blood cholesterol levels, aids digestion and enhances the absorption of nutrients. Also see acidophilus.

Lactobacillus Bifidus

This is a type of 'friendly bacteria' that aids in the synthesis of the B vitamins by creating a healthy intestinal flora.

Lactose

Lactose is a milk sugar. It adds up to about twenty-five per cent of the carbohydrates consumed in an average Western diet. Butter has almost no lactose. Skimmed milk contains more lactose than ordinary full fat milk.

LDL Cholesterol

LDL (low-density-lipoprotein) is known as the 'bad cholesterol'. It's transported to the liver to be broken down and is reabsorbed from the bile into the bloodstream where it could be deposited in the arterial walls. Eat much more soluble fiber, which will bind with cholesterol in bile to prevent such large quantities from being absorbed back into the bloodstream. Soluble fiber is found in beans, lentil, fresh fruit and vegetables.

Lectins

Lectins are plant molecules of non-immune origin that act like powerful antigens. Over a hundred common foods have been shown to have lectins; some are destroyed during cooking, but many are not. Many lectins are poisonous or cause inflammation or both.

Tomatoes have very high levels of these substances, so don't eat too many of them, especially if you have an inflammatory condition. If you have arthritis, avoid them altogether.

Lipids

Lipids are water-insoluble fats.

Lipoprotein

This is a protein bound to a lipid (fat). It aids in the transport of fats around the arterial and lymphatic systems.

Lymph

Lymph is a clear fluid that flows around the lymph vessels, alongside the arterial system. This system is important for collecting debris and unwanted matter from the bloodstream to be removed from the body, as well as carrying nourishment to the tissues.

Lymph Glands (or Nodes)

These are areas where the lymph collects viral, bacterial and waste products for filtering and engulfing by the immune system.

Lymphocyte

A lymphocyte is a type of white blood cell, which forms part of the immune system.

Macro-nutrients

These provide the atoms for structural use in our body, as well as the energy from chemical bonds to power the biochemical processing that continually occurs within our bodies. These macro-nutrients are carbohydrates, proteins and fats. They are needed in large amounts, unlike micro-nutrients.

Malabsorption

This is a term referring to a condition in which the bowel doesn't perform its digestive and absorption tasks properly. Investigations show that malabsorption can occur as a result of any inflammatory condition of the bowel lining.

Micro-nutrients

These are required in small amounts; for example, vitamins and minerals for specific biochemical functions, as opposed to macro-nutrients, which are needed in larger amounts.

Moulds

Moulds are a serious problem. More foods crops worldwide are lost to mould than any other single cause. These substances are often powerful immuno-suppressants. If we become infected they can cause direct and indirect toxic effects. A number of clinical conditions are caused by mould infections, apart from the more obvious athlete's foot and ringworm. These include 'farmer's lungs' caused by moldy hay, 'cheesewasher's lung' from a strain of penicillin, and bagassosis, a condition that affects those working with sugar cane infected with mould. There are about 4,000 moulds that flourish in our homes. Measurements have shown that the average family may give off as much as twenty liters of moisture daily.

Moulds come from many different foods like cheese, mushrooms and bread. Moulds enter via the mouth and can affect the digestive tract, and some people are more susceptible than others. The warm, dark and moist environment of our gut makes a perfect breeding ground for mould to thrive.

MSG (monosodium glutamate)

MSG is processed by glutamic acid, from natural proteins such as seaweed, wheat or tomatoes. The amount found in food naturally is fine, but when concentrated amounts are added to food, it's much too much. On a label, it may be written as 'protein hydrolysate'.

MSG can be found in a huge variety of manufactured foods. Reactions to MSG can range from palpitations, sweating, nausea, headaches, migraines (as in my case), dizziness, etc. Known as 'Chinese Restaurant Syndrome'. If you eat in a Chinese restaurant, check that the chef doesn't use MSG.

Mucilage

Mucilage is a type of fiber, the name describing its texture. Psyllium seeds and linseeds (flax seeds), when added to water, will go slimy and thick, soothing the intestinal lining. A very good intestinal cleanser and stool softener.

Mutagens

These are chemical substances, which can damage the structure of DNA.

Mycotoxins

Mycotoxins are a group of poisonous and often cancer-causing chemicals produced by a number of moulds. Most mycotoxins are only present in tiny amounts, and many appear to pose no threat to us. But a few are deadly, like the potent liver poison and carcinogen aflatoxin B1, secreted by the common mould Aspergillus flavus that grows on wheat, maize, peanuts and other crops. Most mycotoxins survive cooking.

Omega-3

Oily fish is a wonderful source of Omega-3, such as salmon, tuna, sardines, herring and mackerel. These fish are rich in essential oils because of the food they eat, phytoplankton. This oil helps to lower cholesterol, helps to thin the blood and is anti-inflammatory. For those who hate fish, especially the oily ones, there are flaxseeds, also known as linseeds.

Omega-6

Omega-6 is found in sunflower seeds and much more, and is also known as polyunsaturated fat. Omega-6 is readily available, compared to Omega-3, which is generally lacking in most people's diet. However, margarine and many oils are not a good source of polyunsaturated oils. Read the section on margarine and oils.

Omega-9

Omega-9 is found in olives, and is also known as monounsaturated fat. We all know by now how olive oil can protect us from heart disease. Only buy cold pressed or extra virgin olive oil to ensure you get the full benefits of its health giving properties.

Overexposure

Overexposure to a given food or chemical in our diet or environment can irritate and tire our poorly nourished immune cells. Eventually they cause an over-reaction to that food or substance.

Papain

Papain is an enzyme derived from papaya.

Parasites

As many as fifteen per cent of us may be carrying giardia lamblia, a minute flagellated protozoan that causes severe fatigue and bowel disturbance. This is a typical parasite. Parasites may produce illness in several ways. They can undoubtedly produce immune suppression, which will hinder the body's attempt to rid of them. Parasites also compete with your body for nutrients.

Pectin

Pectin is a complex carbohydrate that we are unable to digest, and has an amazing ability to absorb water. It slows down absorption of food, helping to keep our blood sugar levels more even. Also helps to remove unwanted toxins from the body, as well as reducing levels of cholesterol. Found in apples, bananas, cabbage, carrots, peas and several other fruits and vegetables.

Phyto-chemicals

These are substances found in plants that have therapeutic properties.

Phyto-estrogens

Phyto-estrogens are hormone-like fatty acids, derived from plants.

Plaque
Plaque is a build-up of fat, minerals and proteins on arterial walls that can lead to weakening or blockage of a blood vessel.

Polyunsaturated Fats
These are fats from seeds, nuts and vegetables. These oils can easily be damaged or destroyed by heat and processing.

Probiotics
See acidophilus.

Protein
Protein is the major source of nitrogen in the diet. A protein is a large molecule made up of many smaller units called amino acids, some of which are essential.

Prostaglandins
These are hormone-like substances that can promote or prevent inflammation or increase inflammation, depending on the type of food you choose to eat.

Rennin
Rennin is an enzyme used to coagulate protein in cheese-making. Comes from an animal source but there is also a vegetable source.

Shiitake Mushrooms
Shiitake mushrooms contain a polysaccharide - lentinan, which strengthens the immune system by increasing T-cell function. Shiitake mushrooms contain eight amino acids, seven of which are essential amino acids. They are a rich source of B Vitamins, especially B1, B2 and B3. Their effectiveness in treating cancer is well known due to studies carried out in Japan. These mushrooms are also available in a dried form and should be soaked in water for thirty minutes before using them.

Simple Carbohydrates
Simple carbohydrates are found in processed foods that yield simple sugars, which are broken down too rapidly into glucose. The glucose enters our bloodstream too fast and raises our blood sugar levels.

Tannin
Tannin is capable of deactivating a series of enzymes and hindering absorption of certain nutrients, especially iron. Tea is high in tannin. It also has a drying effect. How many cups are you drinking?

Vegetables and Fruits
A National Cancer Institution survey showed that only nine per cent of us eat the recommended five or more servings of fruit and vegetables

daily! Only nine per cent! Some ten per cent of US adults don't eat fruits or vegetables at all in any given day, except fried potatoes.

Villi

Villi are minute finger-like projections found in the intestines, increasing the surface area, which enhances the absorption of nutrients.

Viruses

Viruses are tiny agents that cause infectious disease. They cannot reproduce themselves in the free state, so they seek out a living cell to provide them with both the energy and the chemical building blocks needed for reproduction. Viruses are parasites - once inside our cells they head for the nucleus to try and reorganize the DNA to make the cell's own environment more suitable to their own reproductive needs. If the cells are strong and energetic the 'virus' will have little effect, so the cell's environment remains hostile to them.

Yeast

Yeast is a single-cell organism that may cause infection, given the right set of circumstances.

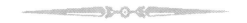

Index

Zambezi Publishing Ltd

We hope you have enjoyed reading this book. The Zambezi range of books includes titles by top level, internationally acknowledged authors on fresh, thought-provoking viewpoints in your favourite subjects. A common thread with all our books is the easy accessibility of content; we have no sleep-inducing tomes, just down-to-earth, easily digestable, credible books.

Please visit our website at www.zampub.com to browse our full range of Mind, Body & Spirit titles, and to see what might spark your interest next...

Our books are available from good bookshops throughout the UK; many are available in the USA, sometimes under different titles and ISBNs used by our USA co-publisher, Sterling Publishing Co, Inc.

Please note:-

Nowadays, no bookshop can hope to carry in stock more than a fraction of the books published each year (over 200,000 new titles were released in the UK last year!). However, most UK bookshops can order and supply our titles swiftly, in no more than a few days. If they say not, that's incorrect.

You can also find all our books on amazon.co.uk, and many on amazon.com. Our website also carries and sells our whole range.

Notes

Notes

Notes

Printed in the United Kingdom
by Lightning Source UK Ltd.
124909UK00001B/475/A